Praise for Deborah
# THINGS I WISH I'D KNOW

*[This] is a strong and much recommended pick for any collection catering to caregivers.*

## Midwest Book Review

*Cornwall has a wealth of knowledge about cancer patients, survivors, and caregivers. . . . [This is] a much-needed support tool for an ever-growing portion of the population.*

## Library Journal

*Cornwall's book addresses everything a caregiver would want to know about. It represents a wonderful balance of compelling first-hand stories and the hard information that new caregivers need to be thinking about early in their journeys. This book provides a tremendous service for anyone facing the challenge of cancer caregiving.*

## Mary Totten
Author, Educator, and
National Healthcare Governance Consultant

*The relatable thoughts and experiences that fill the pages of Ms. Cornwall's book make it a must-read for people who find themselves caregivers as soon as their loved ones utter the words, "I have cancer." . . . Woven together, these stories provide the reader with invaluable resources.*

## Josh Fernandez
Writer and Web Coordinator
Living Beyond Cancer Blog, (LBBC.org)

*As a three-time cancer survivor, I can tell you that the
information and wisdom in* Things I Wish I'd Known *is real
and true. Deborah Cornwall has gathered her insight,
research, and affecting personal stories to provide a book
which itself serves as a comforting companion. It lightens
the load of caregivers so they can minister more attentively
and tenderly to those who must travel the dark and
unknown road of a cancer diagnosis.*

**Joyce Kulhawik**
Emmy Award Winning Arts and Entertainment Critic
President of the Boston Theater Critics Association

*Once I started reading, I could not put down this powerful
book. The stories of the patients and their families are inspiring,
encouraging, informative, and comforting, all at once. This work
has given me new insights about how I should look at our
patients, their families, and their caregivers. Cornwall
completely hits the ball out of the park; this book
will have immeasurable impact on its readers.*

**Paula Baker**
Chief Executive Officer
Freeman Health System, Joplin, Missouri

*Finally a book that deals with all aspects of caregiving for
cancer patients. From the nuts and bolts of patient care and
communication with the medical team to the larger emotional
issues of keeping one's spirits up, sustaining hope, and grieving
when necessary, Deborah Cornwall's book is always to the
point, sensitive, and informative.* Things I Wish I'd Known
*should be among the must-reads of every caregiver.*

**Karla Wheeler**
Founder and President of Quality of Life Publishing Co.
publishers of the hospice quarterly, "Quality of Life Matters"®

*I love this book! It is so practical and real that I know many will be tremendously helped by it. Cornwall addressed every conceivable subject, no matter how sensitive. The two words I would use to describe it are "honest" and "caring."*

**Stephen Swanson**

Past National Board Chair, American Cancer Society, and President of Swanson Consulting LLC

*Cornwall does a masterful job presenting the landscape of the caregiving experience at every stage of the cancer journey in the words of those who have lived it. In the context of relevant, hands-on information and resources that help guide the way, the poignant personal narratives become a true gift and radiate the truth that there really is hope and a path through it all.*

**Bryan Harter, LICSW, MBA**

Former Senior Director, Hope Lodge Program

*Deborah Cornwall takes you through all the steps involved, from diagnosis and treatment to normalcy or life's end, with keen insights and a loving heart. This book is a treasure and will become the caregiver's bible.*

**Barbara Davis**

AstraZeneca Hope Lodge Advisory Board

*This book bolsters the brave, supports the scared, guides the guilty, and helps everyone recognize how hard the caregiver's role is, and how supporting the caregiver supports the patient. I recommend this book without reservation.*

**Joseph Shrand, MD**

Instructor of Psychiatry, Harvard Medical School, Assistant Child Psychiatrist, Massachusetts General Hospital, Medical Director of CASTLE (Clean and Sober Teens Living Empowered).

*As a practicing radiation oncologist and cancer center director,
I see many examples daily of cancer patients, caregivers,
and family needing information and support as they seek
optimal treatment. Cornwall provides a tested road map of options
and considerations to help guide those on a cancer journey.
Her cogent advice covers a host of logistical, practical, medical,
psychosocial, spiritual, and financial domains. These suggestions
should help empower patients and caregivers to actively participate
in information seeking and decision making, thereby enhancing
their role on their own multidisciplinary team. My patients
and families would find it invaluable.*

**Andrew L. Salner, MD FACR**
Director, Helen & Harry Gray Cancer Center,
Hartford Hospital, Hartford, CT
Associate Clinical Professor,
University of Connecticut School of Medicine

*Things I Wish I'd Known: Cancer Caregivers Speak Out is
a valuable guidebook written for the lay person caregiver who
must confront the complexity of the American health care system.
Deborah Cornwall provides a thoughtful and practical guide
through the full range of issues likely to be raised and the problems
to be confronted in these difficult and complicated circumstances.
I think this wonderful handbook will alleviate substantially
the stress experienced by cancer patient caregivers
as they approach their tasks. It's a little jewel!*

**Patricia A. Cahill, Esq.**
Past Chair of the Board of Hope Health

*Cornwall has a firm grasp on the various balancing acts
a caregiver must perform on a daily basis.*

**Phill Powell**
*Touched by Cancer Magazine*

# THINGS
# I WISH
# I'D KNOWN

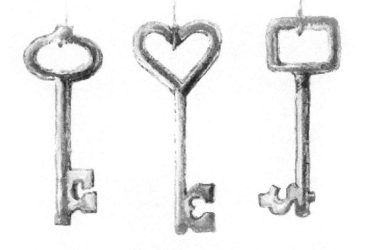

## CANCER CAREGIVERS
## SPEAK OUT

## Deborah J. Cornwall

**Bardolf & Company**
**Sarasota, Florida**

Bardolf & Company

THINGS I WISH I'D KNOWN
Cancer Caregivers Speak Out

ISBN  978-1-938842-27-6

CIP listing applied for.

Published by Bardolf & Company
5430 Colewood Pl.
Sarasota, FL 34232
941-232-0113
www.bardolfandcompany.com

Cover design and layout by Shaw Creative
www.shawcreativegroup.com

Third edition

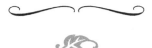

*This book is dedicated to Barry and Debi, who saw me through my own brush with cancer and have continued to support my passion to help find treatments and cures to soften the impact of cancer on others.*

*It is also dedicated to the dozens of caregivers and their loved ones who gave selflessly of their stories, their tears, and their most intimate feelings. Their candor was illuminating as they shared insights they wished they had had when going through their own cancer experiences. Their commitment to the fight, their desire to help others, and their resilience stand as inspirational beacons for all of us who dream about and work toward a world without cancer.*

# Table of Contents

# Preface

........................................................................

Bruce MacDonald

Welcome to Cancerland. You're not sure how you got here. All you know is that it happened in an instant. One minute you were going about your business, living your life, making dinner, calling your mom, planning something for next weekend, and then somebody in a white coat told you or someone you love, "I'm sorry. It's cancer."

Nobody is prepared for this moment. Nobody sees it coming. Nobody.

When you or someone you love is diagnosed with cancer, your whole world is upended. Yesterday's concerns and routines are, at least for the moment, forgotten. Plans for the future, even for next weekend, are put on hold. From this moment on, life in your family will be thought of as "before cancer" and "after cancer." Life as you know it has fundamentally changed.

As an oncology social worker based for the past decade at Dana-Farber Cancer Institute in Boston, I am constantly inspired by the courage and resilience of people like you—patients, family members, caregivers—who are struggling to come to terms with the multiple challenges of cancer. Sometimes it seems like every day brings new questions, unexpected hurdles, and baffling choices. The whole cancer experience, for patients and caregivers alike, can be profoundly disorienting.

So where do you start? In this compelling and practical book, Deborah Cornwall gives you access to a wide range of information, resources, and personal narratives that can truly help you get reoriented. Cornwall teaches you the language of Cancerland by providing the most valuable source of information available: the profound personal experiences and hard-won lessons that cancer caregivers who came before you have learned.

Cornwall's focus is on the roles and responsibilities of the so-called "primary" caregiver—the partner or other individual who is designated to provide the bulk of the frontline support and care. But the truth is, this is a book for everyone involved in a cancer patient's life, including the patient. When someone you love has cancer, you become a caregiver, and there are things you need to know. Deborah Cornwall's book is an excellent place to start.

In "Things I Wish I'd Known: Cancer Caregivers Speak Out," you'll read about spouses, parents, children and friends of patients sharing how they asked the hardest questions, how they faced and made the hardest choices. You'll come to understand that there are no easy, one-size-fits-all solutions. You'll hear people thinking through options, reflecting, debating, second-guessing, searching for answers, and figuring out what it really means to "give care." Ultimately, Cornwall offers something better than advice. In dozens of poignant first-person narratives from people who have been there, she helps you understand how you will get through this. And to believe that you can.

**Bruce MacDonald, LICSW**
Dana-Farber Cancer Institute
Boston, Massachusetts

# Preface
## to the Third Edition

Why, and why now?

The feedback to the first edition, released October 1, 2012, was breathtaking. Readers posted positive reviews on its Amazon.com website. I received emails from caregivers telling me what a reassuring tool it was during their experiences or seeking additional resources. The message from people I didn't yet know, some of whom later became correspondents and friends, was that this book made a difference for them. When someone at my first book event bought the e-book and then came back three times and purchased a total of seven printed copies, I knew there was something special going on!

For me, these experiences reaffirmed that the three-year writing and publishing process—from sourcing interviewees to receiving the first printed copy (which felt like seeing a child being born)—was worthwhile.

Since the book's release, my interaction with cancer caregivers and their loved ones has continued in follow-up interactions with earlier interviewees and in conversations with new caregivers whose compelling stories offered deeper perspectives on what I had written, warranting more attention. People were generous with their suggestions for enriching the content on particular topics by sharing aspects of their experiences that felt most difficult in hindsight.

Nothing has changed structurally or in terms of overall content in this third edition, although all computer links have been updated as of January 2016. Additional revisions and updates include:

- Interviewee demographics have been expanded to incorporate several informal but important interviews. The total is now 101.

◌ The Patient Protection and Affordable Care Act (Obamacare) was under consideration at the time the first edition went to print. The new text reflects the passage of the act into law and the ongoing political pressures about funding it so as to help caregivers figure out how it impacts their situations.

◌ Insights about recent trends in cancer research have been added.

◌ More insights have been woven in about how caregivers heal after caregiving ends, how patients may help caregivers prepare for their death, and the importance of saying good-bye in a permanent form.

◌ Readers are explicitly referred to the resources tab of the book's website, *www.thingsiwishidknown.com*, for newly discovered resources that are specific to particular age groups or kinds of issues. I continue to provide additions in real-time as I encounter them in my travels, since it's impossible to keep them up to date in printed form.

For the most part, this book is timeless. Its issues, lessons, and messages will continue to be relevant to caregivers in the future as they were on the day the words first found their way onto a blank sheet of paper; until we find a way to turn cancer into a chronic disease that you and your loved ones can live with over the long term, with a high quality of life.

May we all live to see that promise become a reality!

**Deborah J. Cornwall**
Marshfield, Massachusetts, January 2016

# Introduction

My own cancer story is far less dramatic than most of those shared in this book. Until my own bout with breast cancer, my only personal cancer experience had come through my mother-in-law, whom I'd known for seven years before marrying her son. She had been fighting metastasized breast cancer for over 15 years, but somehow she always bounced back. Our wedding day was one of her last healthy ones. After the celebration, we settled 350 miles away from her home. We saw her briefly during her last hospitalization, only three months later, but we were emotionally unprepared when she died six weeks after our visit, at age 49. I still cry when I think about how much we all miss her and how much of our lives and her grandchildren's lives she missed. That grief won't quit.

Over the years, as I built my consulting career in corporate leadership and CEO succession, I got involved supporting the American Cancer Society (ACS). I did both volunteer and consulting work and served on several ACS boards of directors. It was intellectually and professionally satisfying work, but I didn't realize for years how far removed it was from the reality of cancer and cancer caregiving. That all changed the day I received my own diagnosis at age 55, exactly 33 years after my mother-in-law's death.

When my doctor told me by phone that I had early-stage breast cancer, I felt like I'd been hit in the gut with a two-by-four. The realization that I had no control over my own health—and was at the mercy of medical professionals whom I didn't yet know, but had to trust—took my breath away. The fact that the surgeon described my cancer as "micro-invasive," and intended to remove lymph nodes as well as the microscopic cancer "lump," was far more terrifying than the subsequent treatment itself.

It turned out that I was luckier than most: The pathology report showed that all of the cancer had come out in the biopsy, surprising both my surgeon and my radiologist. All I had to go through after a lumpectomy was localized radiation, followed by five years of Tamoxifen therapy.

Despite my initial terror, I never felt that my life was at risk. During my radiation therapy, which consisted of 33 mornings of waiting in a hospital gown for the 30-second "zaps," I listened to other women sharing their stories. When I heard a beautiful but bald-headed woman telling another patient about the nine months of chemotherapy she had endured before beginning her radiation, I realized that the definition of a "bad day" was in the eyes of the beholder, and that my own bad days didn't even qualify.

After my treatment, I got more involved with ACS by speaking to various groups in the region and volunteering both in my own community and at Boston's Hope Lodge, which provides free lodging for out-of-town cancer patients. Those activities introduced me to the real, hands-on work that caregivers do in supporting cancer patients. I began to know and interact with people who had lived in the trenches of the cancer battle in ways I couldn't have imagined. I was hearing stories that gave "courage under fire" a new meaning. I began to feel more and more lucky and grateful to have had what I now realize was only a glancing blow from cancer. My appreciation of my own good fortune is what motivated me to write this book.

As I started to interview caregivers, I soon realized that their recollections of the moment of diagnosis in many ways paralleled my own, as a patient with no family cancer history. For instance, Chuck's family had no cancer history when Chuck was diagnosed with metastatic melanoma that had no identifiable primary site. **Chuck's brother**[*] described the family's shock:

> *Cancer is everyone's biggest fear. No one lives in fear of a heart attack, but the word "cancer" is like the word "shark." If someone says the word "barracuda" on a beach, most people would react by saying, "Huh?" But if you hear the word "shark," it triggers a white fear and panic. That's what the word "cancer" is like.*

---

[*] Note: I have bolded references to specific caregivers throughout the book. Many appear a number of times as their testimony relates to various issues.

Most caregivers describe their reactions to a loved one's cancer diagnosis in violent terms: a fast-moving or violent physical assault, a punch in the stomach, a car hitting a deep pothole at high speed, a hijacking, an earthquake, a lightning strike, or a vicious animal bite. A few mentioned a sensation of being frozen and unable to move, or feeling as though a rug had been pulled out from under them.

If you have been suddenly thrust into the caregiver's role, you may have experienced similar sensations when your loved one or close friend received the cancer diagnosis. There's so much information coming from all directions that you may feel overwhelmed, angry, or bewildered. "Normal" has just disappeared from your life. You may be fantasizing that you'll wake up tomorrow and find out that this was all a bad dream. You may even feel resentful: After all, you didn't sign up to set your own life aside to become a caregiver.

Your emotions are real, and confronting them is the first step in coming to grips with your caregiver role. You're probably wondering how this unexpected journey will go, and how it will end. You may be looking for support, guidance, or help—perhaps for the first time in your life—at the same time that you're uncertain where to look, or even what to ask for.

That's another reason why I've written this book.

I networked across the country inviting caregivers to participate in my confidential research and ended up interviewing 101 people and talking informally with dozens more who had "been there and done that." Most of the interviewees were complete strangers to me at the outset of our conversations. Roughly two-thirds of the formal interviews took place by telephone; the rest were done in person, in some cases in the caregivers' homes. I was surprised by the interviewees' eagerness to talk. Most were grateful that someone wanted to listen to their experiences, and all were eager to share what they had learned so future caregivers wouldn't have to reinvent the wheel.

The interviewees came from 19 states and Canada cared for more than 122 family members and friends. Their experiences span 40 different cancers, some quite rare and most life-threatening. Their patients—

children (16), spouses or domestic partners (48), parents and other relatives (27), siblings (10), friends (11)—ranged in age from two to 92. The episodes of care ranged in length from four days to 24 years and counting. Thirteen of the caregivers were cancer survivors themselves.

Roughly half of the caregivers saw their loved ones through to successful remission and a cancer-free life. Others worked their way through terminal diagnoses, treatment to ease physical discomfort, and the process of helping their patients die with dignity and grace. The rest, who still don't know what the outcome will be, are living with the worst kind of ambiguity. No matter what the result, their lives will never be the same.

Regardless of the outcome, these experiences and discoveries have relevance for both caregivers and their patients, and they may help you with your own journey. As **Debbie B's husband** pointed out:

> *There's no better way to learn about dealing with cancer as a caregiver than hearing other people's stories.*

In reading about the key issues you're likely to face and what others did when encountering similar situations, you'll have the opportunity to learn from their approaches and to use them in creating your own solutions to your own unique caregiving challenges. While this book won't serve as a complete "how to" guide or steer you to every resource you might need—caregiving often requires invention under pressure—it will provide guidance and build your confidence in inventing your own way.

Because caregiving requires doing many things at once, there will be occasional repetition as different chapters discuss particular aspects of the process. You may wish to read through the book from beginning to end before going back to the pages that address your unique situation, or you may want to cherry-pick different parts right away. In either case, you'll be broadening your awareness of things to try in response to your own challenges.

Ideally, after reading this book, you'll face fewer surprises and be more ready to fulfill your caregiver role. You may never have been in such an emotionally charged situation before, so as you read, keep in mind what Samantha's mother said: *You're stronger than you think you are. You can do this!*

I was honored that the people I interviewed chose to share their stories and life lessons. Their candor and intimacy were unexpected gifts that enriched my life immeasurably and made this book a reality. In turn, I share their reflections with you in the belief that they will help you on your journey. Their hard-earned insights, their indomitable hope, and their desire to help others to stay focused in the face of adversity represent their way of giving something back to those who helped them.

May you read this book in good health and keep hope alive for your loved one as you navigate the turbulent waters of cancer caregiving.

**Deborah J. Cornwall**
Marshfield, Massachusetts, October 2012,
and updated January 2016

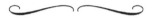

*Why do people love firemen? People love firemen because when everyone else is running out of a burning building, they're running in. It's easier to run away. Caregivers are running into the burning building. Other people care, but they don't know what to do, so they run away.*

**—Chuck's mother**

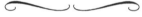

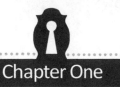

# Chapter One

# What is a Caregiver?

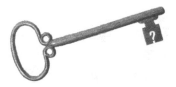

Most people don't choose to be caregivers until a friend or family member requires or requests their support. While the cancer experience is usually traumatic for the patient, it is no less distressing for the caregiver.

The reality is that cancer isn't part of anyone's life plan. Most of us have a vision of what our normal lives could be, and we think we have some control over making it happen. When we're children, we're always looking ahead, to the next birthday or to getting that first precious two-wheeler. As we get older, we look ahead to maybe going to college, or getting our first job, or seeing the world. As adults, we envision broad life stages—developing a career, getting promotions, having a family, and even growing old in relative comfort. These are the kinds of things we daydream about and plan for.

It's no wonder that when cancer hits someone we care about, we're in shock too. It's natural to feel a tidal wave of emotions and a sense of helplessness. The idea that we have control over our lives has just disappeared. As a result, caregivers' recollections of the moment of diagnosis are almost always vivid and photographic. Many describe the event as a surreal, almost out-of-body experience in which they were unable to digest fully the information and events that were happening around them:

**Michael L's mother** *"Cancer" is a taboo word. It never comes into your mind when your child is sick. When they told me, I couldn't see or hear anything. My mind was racing. Mothers want to fix things, but I had to let go.*

**Lynn's husband** *Caregiving happened to me all at once. One night we were having dinner together, and the next morning life just stopped and then everything went in a different direction.*

**Ed's wife** *We had moved to a new state where we had new jobs and no new friends yet. We had come here as an adventure, but it felt like we had gotten on the wrong bus, with only sick people, and we couldn't get off.*

Most interviewees were stunned by the seemingly random nature of the disease. Few of their patients had family histories that pre-disposed them to cancer. Many were young, or athletic and very fit. Almost none were smokers. Most were already eating low-fat diets with lots of fresh fruits and vegetables. Most had kept up with their annual physical exams.

The question "How could this happen?" may never be answered, so once the surprise wears off, caregivers have to be prepared to live with ambiguity. As **Marilyn's radiation technician** counseled her:

*Cancer happens because of a few cells that went crazy. You didn't cause it. It just happens.*

While cancer is an equal-opportunity threat to quality of life and survival itself, there is good news for many: It's no longer an automatic death sentence. That's where caregivers come in.

## What Is a "Family Caregiver"?

If you're working without pay to assist a cancer patient who needs support to pursue the activities of daily life, you are what's called a "family caregiver." (Most family caregivers—87%—are relatives[1], and most of the

---

1 "Valuing the Invaluable: A New Look at the Economic Value of Family Caregiving," AARP Public Policy Institute, Mary Jo Gibson and Ari Houser, 2007, p. 1.

rest are friends.) You're a non-professional who is assuming a pivotal role in helping a cancer patient survive his ordeal with a reasonable quality of life, and you're in good company. Rosalynn Carter, former first lady of the United States, was talking about you when she said, "There are only four kinds of people in this world: Those who have been caregivers, those who are currently caregivers, those who will be caregivers, and those who will need caregivers."[2]

At the broadest level, the National Family Caregivers Association estimated in 2015 that almost 44 million people (over 18% of the U. S. population) provide care for a chronically ill, disabled, or elderly individual during any given year.[3] Cancer is the third most prevalent reason for caregiving, following old age, dementia, and wound care.[4]

More specific to cancer, the American Cancer Society estimated in late 2015 that there were nearly 14.5 million cancer survivors in the United States.[5] This figure doesn't include family members and friends who are taking care of them and may also feel like survivors because the caregiving experience is so taxing. Over 1.6 million people are newly diagnosed with cancer each year[6], and studies estimate that around half of them will be cared for by a member of the immediate family.[7] Even more dramatic is an estimate that 75% of American families will find themselves caring for a cancer patient (relative or friend) at some point in their lives.[8]

---

2 Rosalynn Carter, Remarks as Honorary Chair of Last Acts, *http://gos.sbc.edu/c/carter.html.*

3 *www.thefamilycaregiver.org,* quoting "Caregiving in the United States," National Alliance for Caregiving in collaboration with AARP, November, 2015, p. 4. This study was based on a 2014 survey of 1,248 caregivers. Also, please note that for internet site references within this book, you may need to use the site's search function to locate a referenced topic within the site.

4 Ibid., p. 13.

5 "Cancer Facts and Figures 2014," American Cancer Society, p. 1. Accessible to the public at *www.cancer.org.*

6 Ibid.

7 *www.cancer.org/research/survivaltreatmentresearch/family-caregivers-research.*

8 *www.cancer.gov/cancertopics.*

Family caregivers are very different from professional ones. **Ellen M** was a registered nurse who became a senior executive in a large health care system before being diagnosed with her first brain tumor. Her perspective on caregiving was changed by her own patient experience and that of having her husband as her caregiver:

> *Professional caregivers don't experience the emotional ups and downs that a family caregiver does. The family caregiver truly bears the brunt to support the patient in the right ways, not too much or too little. It's critical for the patient's progress.*

Caregiving takes great strength of character. Sometimes it requires resources you don't realize you have until you carry out this extraordinary role. **Annie's husband** described throwing himself into a heart-wrenching situation as he took over her post-operative clinical care at home for surgical wounds that wouldn't heal:

> *The fact that I could do it for her, be there for her and be the strength that I was supposed to be for her, that's what love is all about. I would have done anything for Annie—anything in the world—and she knew that.*

In some families with multiple children, one child ends up as the primary caregiver when a parent is facing cancer. The other siblings often feel relieved and assume that the primary caregiver will handle the situation, without realizing that the caregiver requires as much support as the patient. For example, **Jack's daughter** had two siblings and a young family, but she ended up as her father's primary caregiver when he was diagnosed with a relapse of prostate cancer:

> *I'm the youngest of three kids. I was 33 at the time and had two daughters, one and three years old. I was a full-time working mom. All of my siblings were nearby, but I became the caregiver, which is a blessing and a curse.*
>
> *My mother had a nervous breakdown while he was declining. She had emotional and psychological problems at the*

*time of the first diagnosis (depression and so on). After Dad's second diagnosis, my sister found her in the shower after she had tried to kill herself. The hospital had us take her home, but she was suicidal so we took turns staying with her. I had no time because I was a working mother and had young kids, so I took leave from my work. I didn't have a choice about taking care of her.*

Part of the caregiving challenge stems from the nature of the disease itself: Cancer is not one disease, but many, and it can be sneaky and unpredictable. According to the National Cancer Institute, there are more than 100 different types of cancer that can arise in nearly any part of the body.[9] All are characterized by cells whose genetic "mother board" is damaged or changed to allow uncontrollable growth that invades normal tissue. The farther the mutated cells travel in the blood or lymphatic systems before settling into a new home, the more complex and challenging the treatment will be, and the more diverse and taxing the demands on both patient and caregiver.

Further complications lie in the toxicity of many therapies and the fact that two patients with the same cancer type may react quite differently to the cancer and its treatment. For some cancers there are "gold standard" treatment regimens with known side effects, while for others the treatments are less proven and available only through clinical trials. For a few, only palliative care (relief of physical discomfort) is possible.

## Prepare to Invent Your Own Way

If you're a new caregiver, you'll face many challenges. You'll need to partner with the members of your medical team while asking questions and, if necessary, pushing back without alienating them. You'll have to be decisive while at the same time giving the patient latitude to control his destiny. You'll seek to restore a sense of control in a seemingly unmanageable situation while going with the flow.

---

9 *www.cancer.gov;* search for "gold standard levels of evidence."

**Bobbi,** a long-time breast cancer survivor, articulated the challenge:

*Caregivers have a difficult emotional role. They don't face the daily adrenaline surge that the patient does, but they have to pick up the pieces when things aren't going well. It's hard for them to know when to reach in and when not to. They walk a tightrope between letting the patient be in control and being able to take care of them without letting their loved one feel incapacitated. Caregivers haven't experienced the physical pain, but they also can't make it go away. The caregiver has to be strong, but not overpowering; sympathetic and optimistic, but not saccharine; realistic but not discouraging; upbeat but not inappropriately happy.*

As you consider playing such a delicate role, you're probably just beginning to figure out what questions you need to ask. Don't be surprised when the more answers you get, the more questions come to mind. Above all, don't expect that your caregiving experience will come in neat sequential steps or that you'll know what to do right away. You may feel like **Tracy's husband:**

*I'd had nothing to help me steer how to behave or what to do. I had to make it up as I went along.*

Your caregiving challenges will vary with the type and severity of the diagnosis. You'll have to wear multiple "hats" as you confront a host of situations:

- ⚜ You could be called upon to shift among such diverse roles as researcher, analyst, secretary, reporter, home health aide, housekeeper, cook, driver, nanny, cheerleader, listener, counselor, project manager, and all-purpose concierge.

- ⚜ In the same day, you might have to change the sheets after your patient has had nausea or diarrhea; help him in and out of the shower, bed, house, or car; help her dress; shop and prepare nourishment; order and pick up medications; care for kids; and take over household responsibilities that your patient can't handle right now.

❧ You may have to manage such treatment-related issues as arranging medical appointments; supporting the patient in making critical medical decisions; reconciling insurance statements against medical bills; overseeing home medication schedules; administering home hydration drips and injections; measuring urine output; changing surgical dressings; tracking and reporting side effects to the clinical team; and keeping the patient comfortable (warm enough, cool enough, hydrated enough, pain-free, and so on).

❧ You're also likely to accompany your patient to medical appointments where you'll be asking questions and taking notes; researching treatment options; tracking the progress of treatments as shown in blood counts and scans; and serving as an information conduit between your patient and his medical team.

At times you'll be bored, and at other times you'll find yourself suddenly overwhelmed with conflicting urgent demands. If you've been a very organized person or a planner in the past, this flurry of unexpected activities will be intensely frustrating.

If all of these varied caregiving responsibilities were put into a single job description, it would be hard to find many candidates who could fit the bill, and the total cost for them would be prohibitive. In fact, the value of such expansive services for all types of caregiving was estimated by the National Family Caregivers Association to total more than $470 billion in 2013.[10]

While the range and intensity of your activities may border on the heroic, don't expect to get a lot of positive feedback along the way. It's not that your patient and his medical team don't recognize or appreciate what you're doing. It's just that they have their hands full, too, and are fully engaged in their own roles. As **Debbie B's husband** said:

---

10 *www.aarp.org.*

*How can you expect someone to be thanking you when she's
sick to her stomach, can't sleep, and is scared to death?*

Know that caregiving will test your physical health, stamina, patience, emotional stability, and commitment to your loved one many times over, and in ways that are hard to imagine. Some days you'll feel so overwhelmed, exhausted and discouraged that you'd like nothing better than to throw in the towel, if only you had that option. This preview of the roller coaster ride and the stresses you'll encounter along the way is not meant to discourage you before you even start on your cancer caregiving journey. Rather, it's intended to encourage you to take a deep breath, summon your inner strength, buckle your seatbelt, and read on with clearer expectations and an open mind.

Many first-time caregivers feel as though they have plunged into a foreign country with a new language, a hostile climate, and challenging terrain. In the words of **Michael L's mother:**

> *You wait your whole life to travel to Italy. Finally, you make
> all the reservations, you collect all the brochures and tour
> guidebooks, and you even learn some of the language. You
> board the plane all excited. When you land, the pilot an-
> nounces, "Welcome to Holland."*
>
> *Shocked, you stutter, "Holland? I'm supposed to be in Italy.
> I have all the guidebooks, the maps, and I even know the
> language."*
>
> *But soon you realize that Holland, too, can be beautiful. It
> has tulips and windmills, and you start to collect new maps
> and to learn a new language. It will never be Italy, but Hol-
> land can be a beautiful place to live.*

She continued to explain that what's important about Holland—her term for the world of caregiving—is that people who've been there will be happy to show you around and may even remind you to admire the tulips. You'll know you're not alone, and you'll be looking at the upside rather than the downside of the trip.

Unlike finding yourself in Holland, your caregiving trip won't be a vacation. Yet if you get the lay of this unfamiliar country, acknowledge and manage your own ever-changing emotional responses, develop your own plan of action, and anticipate the resources you'll need along the way, you will be more likely to make the most of your unexpected journey.

# Chapter Two

# Getting a Clear Diagnosis

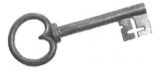

For many caregivers, there is a kind of limbo that precedes the actual cancer caregiving journey. Something doesn't feel quite right with someone close to you; unexplained symptoms persist. You may even be thinking of cancer, but afraid to say it. After all, you never know until there is a definitive diagnosis. It might be a false alarm, which would be the best of news. Often you, as a family member or friend, are called on to provide support during those uncertain times. Whether or not it turns out to be serious, now is the time to begin practicing your caregiving.

It's hard to know what information you need, want, or can handle until you know what the diagnosis is. Getting the diagnosis may seem like something that should be easy and fast, but it's one that taxes the patience of many future cancer patients and caregivers. You'll find that you'll need to demonstrate patience while your physician works to rule out all possible explanations for the patient's symptoms, including cancer,

Interviewees—most of whom were describing very serious cancer cases—cited three major reasons why they felt the diagnostic process happened too slowly:

**Patients Rationalizing Symptoms**

**Standard Diagnostic Protocols**

**Rare Cancers**

Whatever your situation might be, the process of getting the diagnosis right involves your brains, your instincts, and your determination to advocate for your patient. For better or worse, the diagnostic process is also an excellent "training ground," where you can begin to hone your caregiving skills in preparation for things to come.

## Patients Rationalizing Symptoms

For many people who lead busy lives and haven't had a first-hand cancer experience, it's all too easy to put off paying attention to changes in their own or a family member's health. They say they don't have time to go to their primary care physician (PCP) for something that seems insignificant, or they attribute the symptoms to stress, hectic schedules, a prolonged cold, or other transient conditions.

Deep down inside, your loved ones know when something about their health has changed. In some cases, it's their fear of serious medical conditions that causes them to deny the significance of symptoms and to make poor health decisions. If a slight change becomes more pronounced, or if it lasts longer than it should, don't let excuses about a demanding schedule or aversion to doctors and hospitals tempt him to put it off. If he's not feeling right or begins acting strange, and your gut tells you he should consult with a physician, offer to go along, but ensure that he goes.

## Standard Diagnostic Protocols

Many people who do go to see their PCP find that their cancer isn't diagnosed quickly. **Mindy's husband** believes: *Primary care doctors don't look for cancer signs early enough when symptoms don't go away.*

Yet experienced oncologists contend that it's important for them to rule out common ailments first so as to avoid putting the patient through time-consuming, expensive, and potentially frightening tests when they aren't necessary. At the same time, they say that the possibility of cancer should always be considered when the first symptoms don't recede.

**Amelia's husband** felt that her case, which appeared at age 33, was one that her internist missed:

> *Amelia was ill last spring. Then from Thanksgiving through Christmas, she was tired all the time. She went to her PCP several times, but he wasn't doing anything to help her get better.*
>
> *Then she had some seriously abnormal menstrual bleeding and became anemic. She went to her PCP again, and he sent her to the drugstore for iron pills. The bleeding continued, so she cycled through several doctors in the practice until someone recognized that the prolonged bleeding was abnormal and sent her to a cancer specialist, who immediately admitted her to the hospital.*

It turned out that Amelia had serious leukemia. Her husband attributes the delay in diagnosis to our societal attitudes:

> *It feels like Western medicine is symptom-based. You can't go to the doctor and say "I'm tired." He'll give you solutions that seem simple—sleep, exercise, and so on. You don't want to waste the doctor's time, so you wait till you're bleeding.*

Many cancers travel in disguise and can be missed even by high-caliber PCPs. **Herbie's sister**, whose family history with cancer is extensive, says that her brother

> *was misdiagnosed at first by his PCP as having cat scratch fever. Herbie's tonsils were really swollen, so he had them taken out, and they found tumors behind his tonsils. It's still just as devastating every time we hear it.*

The diagnosis was made only after **Herbie's wife** pushed the doctors when the constant tickle in his throat wouldn't go away. Unfortunately, because they didn't know he had cancer before the tonsils were removed, his treatment and recovery have been difficult and prolonged.

Jeff, age 13, was already being treated for chronic asthma when he started to wake up at night sounding stuffed up. According to **Jeff's mother**, a stocky, middle-aged blonde with seemingly boundless energy:

> *The doctors ran lots of allergy tests, and they kept eliminating this and that as the cause. Then he started having night sweats and breathing problems; he'd wake up with his bed soaked. At the beginning of the summer he weighed 83 pounds, and by November he weighed 67 pounds and couldn't keep food down.*
>
> *It was hard to connect the dots because the symptoms seemed random. When I took Jeff to the doctor, our regular physician was out, so we saw one of his associates, who ordered a chest X-ray and blood work. The X-ray technician asked whether Jeff had ever had pneumonia, because he saw a shadow on his lungs.*
>
> *The next day we got a call from his regular doctor asking that we bring Jeff back in and redo the tests. He suspected Hodgkin's or leukemia. He repeated the tests and told us that the situation was serious, so we should see an oncologist. The oncologist did a biopsy of his lymph nodes and lungs. Meanwhile, Jeff was now falling asleep [at school] and at the dinner table, and his lips were blue. When the tests came back, Jeff was diagnosed with stage IV-A Hodgkin's disease.*

Jeff's chronic breathing problems had masked his real illness. Even though he is fine today, he and his mom still remember the drawn-out diagnostic process—it took over six months—with considerable frustration.

There is another reason why some caregivers accuse the diagnostic process of moving too slowly. The medical system and health insurance companies have created protocols that are intended to accelerate the flow of patients through physicians' offices and minimize costs for "unnecessary" tests. Most of us have become so used to the system that we're inclined to go along without complaining.

Yet it's hard to be patient in the face of nagging symptoms. When your instincts tell you that "business as usual" is taking too long without improving the symptoms, or that something is being missed, your job—as a present and future caregiver—is to advocate for your patient and to ask for, or even demand, a referral or a change in the process.

For example, **Michelle's husband** is a tall man with a linebacker's build who is used to making things happen. High standards and a sense of urgency are keys to his professional success as a banker. He had already lost a sister and a brother to cancer when his 36-year-old wife felt a lump in her breast. He described his frustration with today's medical system:

> *Her primary care physician, a young woman, told Michelle that she didn't think it was anything to worry about, even though the lump was large enough to feel. She said to come back in six to eight weeks to have it checked. I was horrified. I think there is a systemic problem with primary care physicians. Their profession is brutally demanding, and they're incentivized not to test the patient. They're paid to manage a file, not a patient.*

Michelle and her husband used his professional connections to get her seen quickly at a specialized breast care center, where she was diagnosed with a five-centimeter tumor in her breast and six metastases into her lymph nodes. Her husband's decision not to accept their PCP's recommendation may have saved Michelle's life.

These examples are not meant to insult primary care physicians— most are hardworking, caring individuals who are themselves under considerable stress and often unrealistic expectations that the doctor will "fix" the patient. Tracy Battaglia, Chief Medical Officer of the American Cancer Society's New England Division, reminds caregivers that medicine is not as black and white as we might like. Primary care physicians, she explains, rely on the prevalence of data to guide their patient workups. While cancer should always be on the list of possibilities, the PCP will generally focus on the more common factors for the patient's particular age and gender group.

However, the caregivers' examples in this chapter do demonstrate that patients and caregivers have the right and the obligation to ask questions if they feel that their physician's actions aren't addressing the core complaint with sufficient thoroughness or urgency. There is nothing wrong with asking the physician whether he has considered the possibility of cancer or some other serious underlying condition. At a minimum, you'll learn something, and at best, you may succeed in accelerating progress.

The bottom line from caregivers is that when symptoms continue despite medical treatment, and you're not comfortable that your physician has gotten to the root of the problem, trust your instincts. For several of the caregivers, it took fresh eyes on the patient—sometimes because the PCP was unavailable or had made a referral—to identify cancer as the cause of the persistent symptoms. As a caregiver, you're entitled to ask questions or or request referral to a specialist to verify that the patient's symptoms are benign.

If that is the outcome, all you've wasted is a little time, energy and money. If it turns out to be something more serious, your shortcut could prove critical in your patient's subsequent treatment and health. So don't stop pushing until you get to the bottom of the symptoms and have a diagnosis that satisfies your mind *and* your instincts

## Rare Cancers

A primary care physician cannot be expected to recognize rare cancers. These generally require attention from specialized cancer centers that support a variety of oncology practices and often maintain their own research laboratories. In many cases, such clinics get involved only when the PCP makes a referral or a caregiver and patient demand answers from the medical system.

The three stories below illustrate the wide range of seemingly common symptoms that can mask rare cancers. The intent isn't to scare you—these cancers are unusual—but to encourage you to keep pursuing the answers you need and deserve about your patient's diagnosis.

**Tim N's wife** described her husband's condition, which began with abdominal pain:

*Tim was 42 years old. In December, he had pain in his abdomen that got so severe that he called his PCP. The doctor said it might be bad gas or a bug and recommended taking antacids. Several days later, Tim felt better.*

*Then, in the spring, he developed a urinary tract infection (UTI). His PCP put him on Cipro and he got better. The UTI came back and Tim was treated with antibiotics three more times. UTIs are very unusual for men, and you don't normally get two or three or four in a row.*

*Finally I called and insisted, "It's been long enough," so he referred Tim to a urologist, who finally in August scheduled a cystoscopy to look at Tim's kidneys and bladder. The urologist said, "You have a fistula* [part of the intestine fused to the bladder], *which is very common for men your age and usually benign." The only way to repair it was surgically. The urologist insisted it wasn't a big deal.*

*The day of Tim's procedure, after four hours, the surgeons hadn't come out. You make all these excuses in your mind about why they were so late, but I was getting nervous. Finally after eight hours, the urologist came out and motioned me to a private room, even though there was no one in the waiting room. I had a horrible feeling. He said, "We went in there and found a mass. We had a pathologist do a frozen section. Tim has cancer. His intestine was tangled around and through the mass and poked into his bladder. We had to remove most of his intestines."*

*Later, after verifying that Tim had a rare form of appendiceal cancer, they said they were totally shocked with what they found. "We were looking for the typical things we see. In a man your age, we're not looking for the zebra."*

**Tim N's wife** had had the strong feeling that something wasn't going right in his nine-month diagnostic process. At every stage, his doctors had spoken confidently about the treatment that they were recommending and Tim's prognosis. Despite all the time that had passed, neither she nor Tim sought a second opinion, and by the time they got a definitive diagnosis, it was too late. She'll never know whether getting a second opinion early on could have saved his life, but as she looks back on it, she wishes she'd acted sooner on her instincts.

For Michael S, a high school student, the trigger was persistent colds and sore throat. **Michael S's father** explained:

> *Michael was a very active senior in high school. During the fall, he had a series of colds and sore throats. We went to the pediatrician, but the physical exam and tests suggested that he was fine. Then at a subsequent checkup, he had swollen glands. The physician gave him antibiotics, and he started to feel better. He was tired, but we just thought he was overly busy.*
>
> *January 1, he was sick again, and we saw him feeling his neck. He could feel something on one side. We decided that my wife or I should go with him to the doctor because this didn't seem to fit the past pattern. Our pediatrician was an older man, but on this occasion he wasn't available. His younger physician partner felt our son's neck and identified right away that it was not swollen glands. He gave us a referral to an ENT specialist, who took a needle biopsy in the office.*

The final diagnosis came in late March from a specialized cancer center, after nearly six months of visits to a variety of medical offices. It was medullary thyroid carcinoma, a cancer so rare that even the specialist who eventually treated him had never seen it in a 17-year-old male. Surgeons ended up removing Michael's thyroid and 100 of his lymph nodes. By following the diagnostic chain to understand why Michael's apparent cold symptoms weren't getting better, Michael's parents found the right treatments and may have saved his life.

Snoring was the action trigger for **Rob's wife:**

> *Three years ago, when Rob was 29, he started snoring out of the blue. It was so bad that the bed shook. After six months, I suggested that he go to the family doctor, who recommended*

*that he have a sleep study done. They diagnosed him with sleep apnea and prescribed that he use a continuous positive airway pressure (CPAP) machine for his breathing while he slept. It was strange that they diagnosed sleep apnea since he hadn't experienced daytime fatigue, but the CPAP helped, so we figured everything was OK.*

*Toward the end of the year, Rob felt a blockage in his left ear. Again we went to the family doctor, and he tested Rob's hearing. He found Rob's hearing was in the low normal range and suggested that we just monitor it. Meanwhile, after one year on the CPAP, now 18 months into the whole diagnostic process, Rob was having worse snoring problems. The doctor suggested another sleep study, and based on the results, he increased the pressure on the CPAP machine's air flow.*

*Nearly two years after the initial medical consult, I started thinking that things just didn't make sense. Rob went to see an ENT, thinking there might be some polyps that needed to be removed. The ENT found a very big mass at the back of his nose and arranged for both a CAT scan and an MRI. These revealed that Rob had an enormous tumor at the back of his nose that was growing around the bones in his skull and wrapping around his carotid artery.*

*After the biopsy, the ENT told us that they had found a tumor and a chocolate-pudding-like substance, saying that he had never seen such a condition before. He sent the sample to a local hospital and then to Johns Hopkins. Two days later, we learned it was a chondroid chordoma, such a rare tumor that only 300 a year are diagnosed in the United States.*

Needless to say, Rob and his wife had traveled a long way from a snoring problem to reach an unexpected and serious diagnosis of Rob's changing situation. The trial and error approach to his diagnosis could have been fatal if she hadn't pushed him to take different action. So far, he has completed his treatment and is doing well despite one recurrence.

In summary, working through the diagnostic tests and waiting for results was the hardest part for many of the caregivers. Some waiting is necessary, and you owe your medical team the opportunity to do a systematic job. Nevertheless, if the symptoms persist or worsen and you don't feel you are making progress, don't apologize for putting pressure on the medical system. If your instincts tell you that the diagnosis and treatment aren't helping, keep pushing to seek more tests, second opinions, or referrals to relevant specialists. Your loved one's life may be at stake, and the minor irritations you're likely to encounter when dealing with the system's perceived inertia are always worth it, whether the results turn out to be benign or serious.

# Chapter Three

# Gathering Information

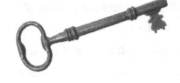

Information represents the first and most critical building block once your patient has received a cancer diagnosis. Bruce MacDonald, LICSW, who has been an oncology social worker with Dana-Farber Cancer Institute in Boston for over 15 years, insists that:

> *There's nothing more important than information in terms of allowing a patient to begin to adjust to and confront what he's facing and to make the most of the rest of his life.*

Information helps you to know what to expect and to ensure your patient is getting the right care on a timely basis from the right people in the right medical setting.

This phase of caregiving is often awkward because you want enough information to be prepared for necessary choices and decisions, but not a flood of data that could drown you and your hopes. This chapter will explore that delicate balance in three sections:

**What Do We Need and Want to Know?**

**Tapping Doctors for Information**

**Using the Internet**

Before you start your search, there is one thing you and your patient should do: Decide how involved each of you wants to be in decisions about treatment. Many of the patients and caregivers in this book wanted to participate intimately at all points. A few, usually older patients or those who are less Internet savvy, preferred that physicians make the decisions.

As a caregiver, it's important for you to talk with your patient early on to find out how involved he would like you to be, recognizing that the more engaged you are, the more help and support you can provide and the more effective you can be as an information conduit with the medical team. Some patients prefer to keep their caregivers somewhat at bay about their emotions and treatment choices. Most of the caregivers who shaped this book, however, were intimately involved in information gathering, analysis of options, and treatment decision-making with their patients.

## What Do We Need and Want to Know?

There's more than enough information in the cancer arena to bury the unfocused caregiver under a mountain of data, so it's important to determine what you want, how much, in what form, and how quickly. Once you know the diagnosis, you'll want to know enough to determine how and where your patient should be treated, and with what objective in mind.

### Decide How Much Information You Want and Can Handle

Some caregivers become information junkies when their gut feelings tell them that something important is being missed in the diagnostic process or that the needs of their loved ones are not being heard by their physicians. Others restrict their information gathering about the particular cancer for fear that the more information they collect, the more difficult it will be to sustain hope in the face of a problematic prognosis; they prefer to focus on the here and now and the next step in treatment, rather than on associated risks and uncertainties.

You may find that you and your patient each need a different "dose" of information at different stages. If so, that divergence needs to be actively managed and communicated. Once you've made that decision, stick to it unless something changes to warrant re-evaluation.

Your job as caregiver and chief information officer is to know how much information is enough for each of you—and how much will be overload. Then communicate those limits to your team.

**Ellen W's husband** handled his and his wife's different orientations to information in a pragmatic way that met everyone's needs:

> *The surgeon came up at the end of the surgery and said, "I'm sorry, it is cancerous. It's a very small spot, but it's definitely colon cancer in the lung." Right then I knew we were dealing with stage IV, so I knew that it was a pretty grim statistic for survival.*
>
> *Ellen really didn't want to know too much about the statistics, but I wanted to know a little bit more. Sometimes we'd meet with the oncologist and she'd leave the room so I could ask some harder questions. Then Ellen could ask me or not. If she was feeling strong enough, she might ask, but it was her choice. Usually she didn't want to know. Each of us needed something different.*
>
> *Through all of this, we can safely say it is a teamwork process, and looking ahead, it's a deeply personal trip we're on together.*

**Tiffany's husband** offered another example of a situation in which a couple had dissimilar information needs. While Tiffany had an appetite for as much information as she could get, he was inclined to take the doctor's recommendation at face value and leave it at that:

> *The oncologist told us to try to avoid the Internet because it would just raise more questions than answers. He wanted to streamline the information we got so we wouldn't confuse or alarm ourselves. He was very business-oriented, but we could always get information. He called her situation one in 350 million as a female diagnosed with colorectal cancer at age 35.*
>
> *Tiffany had been looking up information on the Internet and tended to get upset because she saw that the odds were less than 50%. My role was to slow her down and be the voice*

> *of patience and calm. I had to say to her, "You are unique.
> You're not a statistic."*

Each individual has a different tolerance for medical technical terminology and for survival statistics. Your goal in caregiving is to help your patient to maintain a positive attitude and to remember that statistics only reflect averages and don't predict your own patient's future. Lance Armstrong,
the cyclist whose testicular cancer had metastasized to his brain, was given
a less than 30% chance of survival; yet he beat the odds and went on to
win seven Tour de France bicycle races. His story doesn't mean that every
patient will outlive the averages, but it does mean that you need to interpret
statistics as what they are: a population average. The lead physician is most
able to give you advice about the likelihood of recovery for your patient.

Three examples help illustrate the importance of learning how to use
information for best impact.

**James' wife** is a slender and sharp-featured organizer who has seen
her husband through many years of fighting incurable multiple myeloma.
She used the discouraging initial prognosis to fuel her persistence in seeking out information at every stage of James' illness:

> *I dived in to learn about the disease. It was a rare cancer.
> James asked the doctor how long he'd have, and the doctor
> said a few months if you do nothing, but with a transplant,
> two to three years. So over a long weekend, we developed a
> game plan.*

> *Information empowered me so I could ask good questions
> of the medical team. I felt I was getting better information
> from the doctor when I had that background. Also, James
> was a good patient. He said, "You and the doctors tell me
> what to do."*

> *I faxed a letter from James to the top five doctors in the coun-
> try for his particular cancer. I shared our game plan and
> asked, "What would you do if you were me?" All concurred
> with the recommendations we'd received. Information and a
> clear road map were key for us.*

James' wife has been his chief information officer and project manager during her extended caregiver journey. She stays informed about developments in the field, the newest clinical trials, and where the next step might need to take them. Her dogged pursuit of the most up-to-date information has helped James to treat his cancer like a chronic disease and to overcome the early negative prognosis. He hasn't been without relapses, but her aggressiveness has paid off for both of them. As of this writing, James has lived with his cancer for over 24 years!

**Tracy's husband**, a young, handsome, energetic businessman, has a lot in common with James' wife. When Tracy was diagnosed at age 20 with stage IV Hodgkins Lymphoma, he (as her future husband) wanted to know everything, including the prognosis, so he'd know how to help and how to sustain a positive attitude in the face of an unknown challenge. His recommendation for caregivers is:

> *Do as much research as you can on what you're about to face. Then, after you've processed all of that information, be mentally aware that it's going to be a fight, because your emotions and your thoughts are going to be all over the place. You need to stay positive and understand that as a caregiver, you have to do whatever it is you can do to smooth the ride that this person is about to take.*

> *For us, knowing the prognosis made a difference. We needed for the doctors to tell us that this was something we could come out on top of, and that if we attacked it properly and got her the best treatment available, she was going to be fine.*

Now, at age 40, Tracy holds both an M.D. and a Master of Public Health degree. She is an established internist, public health researcher, and educator specializing in women's health, health disparities, and cancer control and prevention in an inner city hospital. Her patients are thankful for her recovery every day.

Not everyone wants to wade through statistics. Jen P, a mother of two young children under the age of four, had been diagnosed at age 33 with a brain tumor, which was surgically removed from her front temporal lobe. Jen's husband recognized that any statistical prognosis could be inaccurate and even distracting. It helped them as a couple that Jen was in the care of a seasoned physician. They also had young children whose needs distracted them from obsessing about her condition. As **Jen P's husband** explained:

> *We wanted assurances, but no one was giving them. We didn't actively go looking for a prognosis because we realized there's so much that they don't know. Every case is so unique; they're hesitant to give you a prognosis unless they know it's dire and there's not much time.*
>
> *Early on, in a conversation with our surgeon, he said that coming out of med school, you think you know so much, and later on you realize how much you've learned and how much you still don't know. He said "I tell people, 'Live your life in full,' and you can't do that if you take a prognosis too seriously. So much of what we do is science, but so much of it is art, too. You should take every day as it comes, do things you want to do without being foolish, and live your life. "*
>
> *We adopted that attitude and felt good about it and about him. Everyone has issues—arthritis, MS, diabetes—everyone has to deal with something. There's no need to feel sorry for yourself. Just keep moving forward.*

So Jen P and her husband moved on without reams of prognostic data, but armed with a wise oncologist's counsel. Their approach works for them and their young family. There's nothing like a little life wisdom to temper cold, inanimate statistics.

## Block Out Unsolicited Advice

As you go through your caregiving experience, you'll undoubtedly encounter some pseudo-information and unsolicited advice from others. Any number of people may offer unwanted suggestions or make assumptions about what kind of treatment your patient is receiving.

**Artie's daughter-in-law**—a smart, resourceful, and adaptable caregiver—is only one of many who experienced the intrusiveness of unsolicited advice from people who think that if you've seen one cancer, you've seen them all:

> *Not a day went by that someone didn't have some advice for us: You shouldn't be doing this, or shouldn't be doing that. It made me feel incompetent. I just let it go in one ear and out the other. If a person kept pushing, I'd say, "Thanks for bringing that up, we'll check with his doctor." Or I'd shoot my husband a look and he'd intervene.*

Like Artie's daughter-in-law, **Rob's wife** found that it was hard to keep her focus when well-meaning friends tried to offer advice for a complex situation about which they had no knowledge:

> *Some people suggested that we get second and third opinions, but that simply wasn't helpful. The kind of cancer Rob had is so rare, there just aren't that many doctors who know what to do with it. Those people who don't know what to say probably shouldn't say anything.*

Don't let anyone outside your medical circle offer unsolicited information or guidance. It will only confuse or upset you at a time when you need all the confidence you can muster. If they persist, thank them for their good intentions but tell them you only take advice from your medical team.

## Tapping Doctors for Information

Getting your information from a person rather than a computer screen helps to preempt the unnecessary alarm that can result from reading things that may not be directly applicable to your patient's situation. The best physicians bring together a group of professionals on your behalf whose areas of expertise are different but complementary, and they are by far your best resources. The combination of specialists on a medical team allows its members to deal with the whole patient, the patient who is seeking care not only for his physical well-being (length of life), but also for his emotional well-being (quality of life).

Yet the pressures of today's fast-changing health care system are reducing the amount of time doctors can devote to each patient, so it's really important for caregivers to know how to get the best information from your physician as quickly as possible. Your doctor should expect you to ask questions; if he doesn't, find another physician who does.

**Michelle's husband**, the assertive banker, believes that every caregiver should take charge of gathering the information that's needed to help his loved one during the diagnostic and treatment processes:

> *Know the right questions to ask, but don't get bogged down in technical information. Learn the options to consider and the pros and cons of each. 90% of people don't ask enough questions. Don't glaze over when the doctor speaks. Learn enough to know what to ask, when to ask it, and when to push back. It takes a load off the patient if the caregiver will do that.*

This advice is sound. Some of the questions that need answers from your physician and his team are provided in the discussion related to diagnosis and follow-up below. Focus your information search and questions on what treatment will ensure the longest possible life with the highest possible quality of life—comfort, enjoyment and freedom from physical constraints. You will want to know:

- ∽ What is a reasonable goal for treatment? Is this about curing my loved one, controlling the spread or severity of the disease, or just making him comfortable—pain- and symptom-free— for as long as he has?
- ∽ What treatment options are available for this kind of cancer at its current stage? There are often multiple steps in the treatment process, depending on the "stage" or seriousness of the cancer. Primary therapies are used initially after diagnosis and may include surgery, radiation, chemotherapy, or any combination of the three. Subsequent treatments, known as adjuvant therapies,

are used after the initial course of treatment has been complet-ed. When considering treatment options, you should be asking:

- Surgical recovery: How long will it take? What kinds of complications or potential setbacks should we anticipate?

- Returning to the hospital: What kinds of situations should bring us back to the hospital for treatment? Whom should we contact in such a situation in order to get treatment quickly?

- Potential side effects: What should we expect during treatment? How might we best handle them to miti-gate stress? Every patient reacts differently to each kind of treatment, but general information about common patterns can help you anticipate and manage their ef-fect on your patient.

- Impact on daily living: How is the recommended course of treatment likely to affect work schedule, availability/ ability to handle household tasks, and so on?

- Other medical conditions: How will the recommend-ed course of treatment affect other medical conditions for which the patient is currently being treated?

✍ How urgent is it to start treatment? The more aggressive the cancer, the more important it may be to start treatment right away. The diagnosis is generally confirmed by a biopsy, which involves extracting a sample of the patient's cells and sending them for testing and examination by a pathologist.[11] The pa-thology report often includes a cell "grade," which indicates the level of aggressiveness—the speed with which a tumor will grow and invade surrounding tissues or systems—and the relative urgency of getting treatment. For solid tumors,

---

11 Pathologists are medical doctors who specialize in the prevention, early detection, and diagnosis of cancer and other diseases. They examine tissues and fluids to diagnose disease in order to assist in making treatment decisions. For more information about pathologists and biopsies, see *www.cap.org*.

39

severity is generally measured in terms of stage and/or grade. Higher numbers are more serious than lower ones. The pathology report and the individual doctor's experience with the particular kind of cancer generally determine how much time you have to seek out information and even second opinions. (See Chapter Four: Choosing Treatment Partners.)

Most physicians are able to recite statistics about average survival rates for particular cancers at any given stage. Yet they will also keep reminding you that your patient is an individual whose unique situation isn't predefined within statistical boundaries. They tend to recommend that you draw on them for your information about the progression of the disease because, as explained above, they don't want you to be alarmed by statistics or negative stories that don't necessarily reflect your patient's condition. At the same time, the best physicians understand and support the caregiver's intense need for more information.

**Mike S's wife**, a soft-spoken but determined advocate for her husband, refused to accept the four- to six-week estimated survival time that accompanied his pancreatic cancer diagnosis. She began researching clinical trials at the outset, long before the Internet was a readily available information resource:

> *I became an information wonk. Mike's oncologist was very supportive. He even requested that Mike be the last patient of the day so he could spend time with us. I was calling doctors all the time. I prepared questions and asked about treatment options. When I learned about a clinical trial, I would contact the principal investigator, and I was gratified when they would take the call or call back quickly.*

> *At one point, while we were waiting to see our doctor at the end of the day, I asked Mike if my crazy research was embarrassing or annoying or exhausting him. He said, "No, it gives me courage." He wanted options. My "research" just helped us feel in control. I never brought up a clinical trial that our oncologist didn't know about.*

Because of her networking to find more information and more clinical trials that might work for Mike, his wife succeeded in extending his life more than two years beyond the original prognosis.

Talking directly with the physician is most appropriate but doesn't always provide a clear message. Many cancer caregivers and their patients want so much to receive encouraging news, that sometimes they hear only what they want to hear. **Bruce MacDonald** explained this phenomenon:

> *Even a physician who does present information in a clear and kind way can still be grossly misinterpreted by a patient. He may say, "We cannot cure this cancer, but we can treat it." And the patient comes away thinking, "Thank goodness they can treat it (and I'll come through this fine)," and misses the message that he may not survive his cancer.*

**Tim N's wife** looks back on his diagnostic and treatment processes and feels that she may have heard what she wanted to hear when "doctor-speak" gave her room for denial:

> *It never crossed my mind that he'd die, even when he got really sick. It's clear now that I should have known much earlier. When his doctor said the odds were 50/50 for the next treatment to be effective, we heard that to mean there was some chance they'll cure you.*
>
> *I felt angry afterwards. I felt cheated. I really trusted them. When the doctor told us of the recurrence, he had a smile on his face. I translated that to mean that it can't be so bad because he's smiling. They'll find something that works because he's smiling. I didn't realize that he was smiling because he was sheepish and didn't know what else to do or how to deliver the news.*

She might have asked for clarification, but perhaps not asking left room for her to believe he would survive.

According to **Bruce MacDonald**, some of the challenge in deciphering "doctor-speak" comes from the fact that information provided by surgeons isn't necessarily delivered with the sensitivity that you might experience from other types of oncology physicians:

> *Surgeons in my experience are notorious for telling people, "We got it." They don't want to deal with the patient's affect and reaction to hearing the news that the cancer is widespread or metastatic.*

> *Remember that surgeons have little contact with patients when they're awake. It's a fairly self-selecting crew. A good surgeon is brilliant with a knife and brilliant with a team. His bailiwick isn't understanding the arc of an illness and what will help a patient cope. Sometimes you may want to believe that surgical treatment is your encounter with God and that your life is in the surgeon's hands, so you don't want to believe he's fallible or not all-knowing. It's important for people who read a book like this to know that.*

Several interviewees validated his perspective by describing their stunned reactions when their cancers returned after they had heard a "we-got-it" assessment from their surgeons. The reality is that despite our trust in doctors, it's impossible for a surgeon to predict whether a particular cancer will return or not, and each doctor has his own style and bedside manner. Your challenge is to find one whose manner matches your patient's needs.

Sometimes a physician may hesitate to offer a recommendation when you ask a question about treatment options. If this happens, try asking him, "What would you suggest if the patient were your wife, husband, child, or parent?" Often this question will extract a recommendation that the physician would otherwise be hesitant to offer. The decision on which option to choose is ultimately the patient's, usually in consultation with the caregiver, but the physician's answer usually says a lot about which one is most likely to meet the patient's goals.

There are situations, though, in which seeking information from physicians and managing expectations can be a no-win proposition for everyone concerned, as **Debbie B's husband** explained:

*With appendiceal cancer, it's not if the patient will die, it's when. It came down to whom do I trust? How much do I need? Do I trust the medical team? We had decided to work with this doctor and this institution unless something felt like it was going really wrong. We weren't going to second-guess what the doctors said.*

*After Debbie's first surgery, we lulled ourselves into thinking she had this thing beat. We didn't do enough research to understand what kind of cancer she had. She felt well. Her scans were coming out clean. We didn't want to ask, "Will it come back?, or when." Time passes, and you just think things will be OK.*

*When you have a disease under the cancer umbrella that's almost certainly fatal, what does more information give you? The goal here is quality of life and longevity, and a balance of those two. The balance between quality of life and longevity differs by the person.*

In treating Debbie B, the physicians and her caregiver were stuck between a rock and a hard place, telling the hard-edged truth while still sustaining hope.

## Using the Internet

The Internet poses a special challenge. It's a blessing because voluminous information can be accessed quickly, but it can also become a curse when it threatens to overwhelm you with data. The Internet is a little like a fire hose: if you're a little thirsty, it's difficult to get just a sip of water, so plan carefully before you turn it on. **Bruce MacDonald** put information-gathering on the Internet in perspective:

*You get the good, the bad, and the ugly on the Internet. Once in a while, there's actually something of use, like a particular trial. It doesn't happen that often because most of the professionals in cancer centers are in touch with people around the world and are researchers themselves, so they know what's happening.*

43

Using the Internet effectively requires focus and self-discipline to avoid conflicting sources and confusion, or drowning in alarming or negative information. The most common messages about the Internet from the interviewees are: Know what you're looking for, make sure you're reading reputable sources, and get out before you're tempted to get into a level of detail that you've already decided you didn't want. They had three specific recommendations.

## Focus Internet Reading and Test Findings

**Patti's daughter** found that a careful and focused Internet search—preceded and followed by reality checks with the medical team—eased her sense of powerlessness:

> *As a caregiver, you'll feel helpless, and you'll want to fix this. So get informed, and don't just accept that the doctor doesn't know. Just a Google search gives you crap, so we got information from the oncology doctors and nurses to get the actual medical terminology that they use so I could research on that and not just cancer or lung cancer. Then I did online research with WebMD and the American Cancer Society.*
>
> *I read everything I could get my hands on. I had the doctors on speed dial for clarifications on information that I gathered. I used to joke with one of the doctors that I probably called him more often than his wife did.*

If you decide to use the Internet, focus your search on trustworthy information from reputable medical sources. Several cancer-focused and hospital-based websites can provide you with responsible and easily usable information about both cancer in general and specific types of cancer:

- ᠊ᓭ The American Society of Clinical Oncology (ASCO) (*www.cancer.net*)
- ᠊ᓭ The American Cancer Society (*www.cancer.org*)
- ᠊ᓭ The Association of Cancer Online Resources (*www2.ACOR.org*).

❧ CancerCare *(www.cancercare.org)*.

❧ National Cancer Institute of the U.S. National Institutes of Health *(www.cancer.gov)*. At this website, it is possible to get a list of NCI-designated cancer centers *(www.cancer.gov)* and enter "cancer centers" into the search function.

Your goal should be to identify leading hospitals and physicians that have intensive experience with your patient's particular type of cancer.[12] In addition, there are many foundations or associations that offer information about specific types of cancer. If you enter your type of cancer into an Internet search engine, it will bring up a number of such organizations. Information they provide can be particularly useful for providing less-involved family members or friends with a common information source.

## Use the Internet for Fast Access when Time is Precious

For patients whose prognosis is desperately grim or who are participating in clinical trials,[13] time is of the essence. In these cases, the Internet can be a wonderful tool to accelerate critical conversations with the medical team.

Easy access was helpful to **Doug's mother**, who used the Internet to "get smart fast" when her 14-year-old son was being treated for Ewing's sarcoma. Although she was an experienced senior corporate executive, she found the amount of available information overwhelming at first, in part because Doug's cancer was so serious. With time she found that it helped her interact more successfully with the medical team because she could ask better questions:

> *We were in shell shock, so I went on the Internet and read everything I could find. Most of the information said it was*

---

12  A particularly good resource for guiding you in what questions to ask of your own physician and potential specialists is Ellen Menard's "The Not So Patient Advocate: How to Get the Health Care You Need Without Fear or Frustration," Bardolf & Company, Sarasota, FL, 2009. See particularly Chapter Four, "Dealing with Specialists," p. 76-80.

13  The topic of clinical trials is addressed in Chapter Five.

*highly unpredictable and gave a negative prognosis. My first reaction was "OMIGOD, my kid's going to die." Then you think about how much medicine has changed, and it won't happen to us because we'll have a miracle. It was a balancing act, because you really need hope. Once we had the context from the web, it helped us understand what the doctors said.*

**Rob's wife** went on the Internet with her eyes open after the cause of his severe snoring was finally diagnosed as chondroid chordoma. She deliberately sorted through the negative stories to find hopeful pieces of information. Sharing one of them with Rob's oncologist helped them to assemble the right medical team to treat his rare cancer:

*I got back on Google, but I wasn't sure I wanted to do this. Everything I saw was all bad, but I needed to see that people have survived this kind of tumor. In my research on the Internet, I located the Chordoma Foundation. There were lots of stories there, and information about surgical options, but it was clear that you needed the right surgeon and that radiation would require proton beam therapy.*

*The local oncologist had never heard of it and said "I can't do it, but don't give up." When I shared with him what I had learned on the Internet, he went on the website for the Chordoma Foundation and made contact with an oncologist, who referred me to a nearby radiation oncologist who had worked at Massachusetts General Hospital. This doctor showed us the scans and explained that he had treated these kinds of tumors before. He got the ball rolling and referred us to a third oncologist at Mass General for the radiation. Being in limbo was not as bad now because at least we knew that the right person was developing a plan for treatment.*

Carefully targeted Internet searches, framed by physicians at the outset or tested with them afterward, can be useful for patients and caregivers who want more information than doctors have time to provide. They are particularly helpful in finding scarce resources for treating "zebras," the kind of urgent rare cancers mentioned in Tim N's story earlier.

For many caregivers, getting the right kind of information also allows them to regain some control over a situation that feels like a helter-skelter free fall. **Sharon's sister** found Internet information calming both when her young niece was in leukemia treatment and again when Sharon was diagnosed with aggressive breast cancer at age 38. She understands the value of having quick and comprehensive access to information when you're feeling overwhelmed:

> The Internet helped me process in an organized way. It's great as long as you realize that you can't trust it all. I had specific questions, and it was wonderful to have right at my fingertips a way to immediately get an answer. It helped me to focus on what we could do and made me feel I can do something right now.

### Use caution before accepting predictive statistics

Some Internet sites present survival and prognosis statistics without providing interpretive context. That may lead to misunderstandings regarding their relevance to your situation. According to **Bill P's wife:**

> The Internet misleads you about statistics. When they say something isn't a problem for 70% to 80% of people, they don't tell you that they're looking at the entirety of the population. For example, those who get prostate cancer are older and generally are suffering from other problems and die of something else, so general statistics about prostate cancer don't take into consideration how old your patient is.

It's imperative to remember that the Internet is far less useful in determining the prognosis for your loved one than your own medical team, which will present information in context.

In conclusion, information is your road map. It's a critical tool. You need it not just at the outset of your cancer journey, but throughout the trip, to verify where you are and to plot out where you're headed. At each pivotal stage, you'll develop more questions and need more answers, or perhaps answers of different types. You'll be broadening out your data sources and calling on more resources to meet your needs. As you learn more, you'll ask smarter and deeper questions, and you'll be ready to absorb more nuanced information. You will have grown wiser, more discerning, and more focused in your search, and you'll be that much more helpful to your patient.

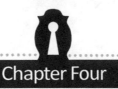

# Chapter Four

# Choosing Treatment Partners

If you knew you were about to land in a foreign country, wouldn't you like to have a knowledgeable guide to tell you where to go and what to avoid? The difference with being dropped into the cancer caregiving world is that the choices on your journey have significant quality and length-of-life implications. Once you get a cancer diagnosis, you and your patient will need guides to help you decide on the course of treatment and who will provide it. While every cancer patient hopes for the best—a short and survivable cancer episode—your partnership with various members of the medical community may be long-lasting, so you'll want to get it right from the start.

This chapter will cover five broad topics to help you know what questions to ask as you go about making these decisions:

**Selecting Your Medical Team**

**Community Hospital vs. Major Cancer Center**

**Referrals, Networking, and Cold Calls**

**Second Opinions**

**Switching Physicians or Hospitals**

## Selecting Your Medical Team

For your cancer journey, you will want to assemble the *right* medical team that is most likely to provide the best possible outcome. "Right" includes not only correct and effective medical care, but also care for the whole patient, including his quality of life and emotional needs, and respect for the caregiver as an integral part of the team. Above all, "right" means getting a team leader whose judgment you trust and with whom you feel comfortable having candid and constructive discussions about treatment options and outcomes.

**Ellen M's husband** described what makes a good partnership with a medical team and its lead physician:

> *We really like her oncologist as a person and as a professional. He is a warm person and he will always tell you what he knows. He doesn't like to conjecture, but sometimes we have to ask him to do so. If I put myself in his shoes, I'd deal with us as he does. He doesn't spout statistics, but if we asked, he'd tell us. We've had nothing happen that made us say, "Why did they do that?" or made us feel we had to watch them every minute. We poke and prod a little bit when we feel the doctor needs to tell us more, but he always gives us answers that are smart and caring.*

Smart *and* caring. It's clear that Ellen and her husband did well in selecting their medical team. If you go over Ellen's husband's description carefully, you'll see that he is describing both the quality of medical care the oncologist delivers and the ways in which he interacts with them. As you read on, you'll see references below to a doctor's technical competence as the "hard facts" and to his interactions with his patient as "chemistry."

### First Consider the Hard Facts

The first thing you'll want to get smart about is the medical aspects of care, the "hard facts." In general, dealing with cancer requires a group of medical professionals working together to bring the best possible outcome for each patient. Among the reliable professional resources for gathering enough information to frame your decision are:

- ᷤ The American Cancer Society (*www.cancer.org*), 800-ACS-2345

- ᷤ The American Society of Clinical Oncology (*www.cancer.net*), 888-651-3038. This organization has instituted a Quality Oncology Practice Initiative (QOPI) which certifies medical oncology and hematology/oncology practices for meeting high standards of patient care and safety. Ask about this certification if you will be receiving chemotherapy infusions.

- ᷤ National Cancer Institute at the U.S. National Institutes of Health (*www.cancer.gov*), 800-4-CANCER (800-422-6237)

Each of these organizations has a website that provides guidance regarding the kinds of medical professionals who may be involved in your patient's treatment, how to select your medical team, and how to choose a hospital. All explain what different health professionals do and what questions you'll want to ask before signing on with a particular doctor or hospital. All emphasize that the physician you select should meet the following seven standards:

1. **Credentials:** Hold the appropriate degrees (generally M.D. or D.O.), have completed the requisite practical training (internships, residencies, and so on), and be licensed to practice. If he is a specialist, he should have had one or more years of additional training, have earned "fellowship" status in his appropriate specialty society (such as medical oncology, surgical oncology, hematology, and so on), and be board-certified in his fields. (You can check on any doctor's certifications at *www.abms.org*, the American Board of Medical Specialties.)

2. **Experience with this particular diagnosis:** Have extensive experience in the field and treat a significant number of patients

with this particular diagnosis on a regular basis. (Unless the cancer in question is exceedingly rare, you don't want the doctor learning on your patient.)

Some doctors treat patients, teach, and do research to help advance understanding of how various treatments influence outcomes for different types of patients. These doctors often publish papers outlining their findings and highlighting key areas of their expertise.

3. **Expert hospital affiliation:** Practice at a hospital that is certified by an independent hospital accreditation body, such as the Joint Commission (*www.jointcommission.org*) or the Healthcare Facilities Accreditation Program (*www.HFAP.org*). The hospital should also have a reputation for high quality care and a successful track record in treating the patient's specific cancer type. Such certifications refer to the overall quality of the institution but not necessarily to cancer care.

   Different cancer centers are known as centers of excellence (a term reflecting a concentration of expert resources) for different specialized forms of the disease. In addition, a cancer center that is associated with a medical school or maintains its own research facility may represent an especially good choice for less common cancers. (More specialized accreditation for more sophisticated cancer centers is addressed later in this chapter.)

4. **Multidisciplinary team play:** Cooperates well with other physicians and support resources to ensure that you get the most complete care possible. Is willing to share information to streamline your patient's care and provide you with copies of lab results and files. Also answers questions constructively, and is comfortable to:

   • Ask questions and engage in dialogue on the full range of issues affecting your loved one's care.

   • Solicit a second opinion from other specialists.

- Ask what other research resources will be most useful.
- Test what you learn from outside resources, including the Internet, with your doctor.
- Accompany your patient to every appointment.
- Take notes or record the session as a resource to help the patient.

5. **Insurance:** Accept the patient's form of insurance.

6. **Language:** Have appropriate translation services available if the family has a multicultural background.

7. **Back-ups:** Have other expert physicians covering for him when he is not available. Work with a multidisciplinary team that has experience in sharing information and providing information and care to the patient as required when unexpected setbacks occur.

This last item is critical. You have no idea when your patient will experience some sort of adverse reaction to a procedure or treatment, and you need access to good medical coverage 24 hours a day, seven days a week. Your physician is human and needs time off, but a truly professional doctor will have someone covering for him at all times, as well as good systems in place to ensure that he is notified personally when critical problems arise.

## Then Consider Chemistry

In addition to the "hard facts," you'll find that chemistry, a softer and more subjective variable, is just as important in selecting a physician and the medical team. You want to ensure that the team will be sensitive to the stresses that both patient and caregiver are experiencing. Good chemistry means that you feel you can have unqualified trust in the doctor's judgment and advice, engage in a comfortable two-way flow of ideas, and get a sense of realistic hope. It also means having full confidence that all of his team members have your patient's physical and emotional well-being as their goals.

Many of the caregivers interviewed for this book found physicians who combined a high level of expertise with an approach toward care that encouraged patients to be advocates on their own behalf.[14] In the words of **Carole's husband**:

> *You need the relationship to be extremely warm and fuzzy. Then it's easier for you to feel comfortable being an advocate and asking personal questions. It was extremely important that the doctor we worked with was able to hear what we wanted to say. There were plenty of doctors we met who would push back or be somehow condescending if you asked a question or if you said, "Hey, what do you think of this?" We used to go in with pages of questions about things we had read about. The people we chose would sit and tell us what they knew about them.*

Jen P's and her husband's choice of oncologist was also based on a combination of expertise, approach, and comfort level after her MRI revealed the encapsulated tumor in her front temporal lobe. As **Jen P's husband** describes it:

> *We opted against doing a biopsy and chose to get it out right away. To consider who should do the surgery, we checked out three leading hospitals, two of them out of town, and got the same diagnosis from all three. One of the surgeons was going to be more aggressive with his approach than we were comfortable with. We thought with the brain, let's be careful and get as much as we can with certainty, and then treat the rest with radiation.*
>
> *We fell in love with the surgeon at the local hospital. He was in his last year of work. He was comforting, almost father-like. I was 36 at the time. His style felt almost like my dad's. He was cautious and calming. I'd see things on the Web that made me go OMIGOD, and he was a good sounding board who could calm me down.*

---

14  The role of being an advocate for a patient is addressed in Chapter Six, p 90.

This surgeon described to Jen and her husband how he had drifted into administration at another prestigious cancer center but soon decided that administration wasn't why he'd gone to medical school. When he told them that the last 12 years had been the best of his career, because he was head of neurosurgery and working directly to treat patients, they knew he was the right surgeon for them.

Other caregivers and patients describe the importance of chemistry in the relationship with their principal cancer physician. For **Darcy's husband**, it was the surgeon's brilliance, breadth, and style:

> *We got the head of the surgical team, who happened to be 32 and had already written books on cooking for cancer patients. He was like a renaissance man. He'd had a triple major in college: math, biology, and Russian art. He also had a great personality and bedside manner. A brilliant guy. An unbelievable personality. He wasn't your typical arrogant surgeon.*

For **Mike S's wife**, it was his oncologist's unexpected candor and compassion:

> *When I first heard about this surgery, I was beside myself. One day, I went to talk to our medical oncologist about it. I didn't have an appointment, but I just marched through the halls until I found the poor man in a little office working at his computer. I plunked myself down and told him I was terrified. He replied, "So am I."*
>
> *Of all the answers in the world, that was the right answer for me. He responded from his gut and his heart. He acknowledged my panic and pain. Then he went on to say that he had researched the options, the surgery, the surgeon, the hospital, and he was convinced we were doing the best thing, with the best surgeon, at the right hospital. That gave me hope.*

There is no one right answer for how to balance the hard and soft criteria, as long as you don't have unrealistic expectations that a surgeon, who isn't necessarily trained to be sensitive, will be sympathetic and caring, or that the right medical team can produce a miracle for your patient. The appropriate balance of hard skills and relationship skills is likely to vary by professional discipline, so be sure you recognize where you need the full package and where technical skills alone will best meet your needs.

When push comes to shove, you need the surgeon to be technically superior in skills and experience, regardless of his bedside manner. That drove **George's daughter's** choice:

> *When we made decisions about medical staff, our attitude was for surgery, get the best surgeon. We didn't care about bedside manner (whether my father and he got along). We also learned that in oncology, you don't know what will work until you start it. So you'd rather have a medical oncologist who was attentive and would meet with him more often to adjust the dosages based on his reactions.*

If your surgeon turns out to be that special balanced kind of person, so much the better, but if not, you may need to seek the compassionate side from your medical and radiation oncologists.

## Community Hospital vs. Major Cancer Center

One topic on which most caregivers agreed is on the choice between a community hospital and a major cancer center. Not every cancer requires a sophisticated cancer center's resources or level of specialized expertise. Yet their recommendation: If you have a choice, trade up, at least for a second opinion to ensure that your local hospital is giving you the best recommended course of treatment. **Michelle's husband** put it very directly:

> *The first crack at the cancer is always your best chance. Don't necessarily stay in the local community. Get to a major cancer center. Go online. Get in the car. Use every resource you can. Be an aggressive firefighter. Get enough education that you can be an aggressive health care consumer. Insist on getting heard and advocate hard without getting thrown out of the room.*

**Bill**, a prostate cancer patient, added:

> *Your best bet is the major cancer centers. There, every case is reviewed with multiple doctors from multiple disciplines, so you have a higher probability of a better solution.*

Most patients who switched doctors or hospitals were changing from a community hospital to a more sophisticated cancer center or oncologist. The only exceptions were patients whose initial treatment occurred at a major cancer center a long way from home and who chose to have the chemotherapy prescribed by that center but administered closer to home.

Caregivers insist, however, that you not quibble over travel distances for any service that may have life-or-death implications. **Abby's sister** says that their long travel was worthwhile:

> *Every hospital is suddenly calling itself a cancer center, but many are just local hospitals that have oncologists and new signs. The city research hospital has a team of doctors and support staff for different types of cancers. It's clearly different from the moment you walk in. The doctors are researchers and are going for all the cures they can get. They had our kind of attitude, so we took them onto our team. Their goal was for her to live with an excellent quality of life.*

She and others advise going for the best, and then, if necessary, seeking out available free or discounted lodging options (as outlined in Chapter Seven, page 117) or free rides to treatment (800-ACS-2345) if necessary.

One way to evaluate a potential hospital is by its accreditation. The American College of Surgeons maintains a Commission on Cancer (CoC), which describes itself as "a consortium of professional organizations dedicated to improving survival and quality of life for cancer patients through standard-setting, prevention, research, education, and the monitoring of comprehensive quality care." A medical care facility accredited by the CoC has achieved high standards in a variety of parameters, including:

- ৵ Quality care
- ৵ State-of-the-art services and equipment
- ৵ Multidisciplinary care
- ৵ Access to appropriate information and support
- ৵ Ongoing monitoring of care
- ৵ Information about clinical trials and new potential treatments
- ৵ Maintenance of a cancer registry that tracks patients from the initial diagnosis through the rest of their lives to help improve diagnoses and treatments for others

Only about 1,600 of the 5,700 hospitals registered by the American Hospital Association are CoC-accredited. Such accreditation is one indicator that a facility is providing competent and trustworthy cancer care. To receive accreditation, a cancer center must provide state-of-the-art pre-treatment diagnosis, treatment, and clinical follow-up, led by a cancer committee that oversees quality and works to improve patient care. In addition, the center is expected to conduct cancer conferences, contribute to physician education, and participate in appropriate geographic cancer registries to monitor the quality care as a foundation for evaluating and improving patient outcomes.[15]

A further and more important certification comes from the National Cancer Institute (NCI), which (as of January 1, 2016) has designated 68 cancer centers in 35 states and the District of Columbia that support care for patients with intensive laboratory and clinical trial research. Of these, 45 are designated as Comprehensive Cancer Centers because they offer broad clinical cancer care, support research to advance new treatments, and encourage both transdisciplinary research and clinical trials. Comprehensive Cancer Centers are often associated with medical schools and complement clinical care with research and clinical trials, often in cooperation with other such centers. Seventeen hospitals are NCI-designated as Cancer Centers; and seven, as Basic Laboratory Cancer Centers. Data on

---

15 *www.cancercenters.cancer.gov.*

treatment efficacy and patient outcomes are increasingly shared among these institutions, together with best practices in patient care.

The range in types of certification (from the most sophisticated Comprehensive Cancer Centers to Community Cancer Centers) allows people living in more rural areas to access higher quality cancer care for portions of their treatment as needed.

Be cautious in considering a for-profit hospital that makes success-rate promises for advanced cancers that sound too good to be true. They usually reflect selectivity in the cases and insurance situations they are willing to accept, so that their statistics aren't comparable to national or non-profit hospitals' statistics. If it sounds too good to be true, it probably is.

## Referrals, Networking, and Cold Calls

If you know any people in the medical field, they are likely to know other people who have contacts who can help you get to the right places within the health care system. Don't hesitate to network that way. You may be surprised by the number of people who would be happy to help you find the right medical team. **Michael S's father** got the referral directly:

> It was a whirlwind. Within a week, we were in at the right hospital with a physician who had been a classmate of our primary care physician. Our PCP had called ahead to grease the skids. Calling cold for an appointment would have taken six months with this particular physician.

**Darcy's husband** used personal networking:

> My daughter worked in a bank and got a bank board member to contact a board member at the cancer center we chose, who put us in contact with the head of oncology, whose reputation was outstanding.

If you don't have connections you can use, don't worry. Since **Michelle's husband** had lost two siblings to cancer, he wasted no time finding his wife the best possible breast cancer care, even though he didn't have direct contacts in the medical profession:

*I learned of a physician who had been director of breast cancer and research at one of the three best hospitals. He was the point person for a new collaboration among the three hospitals I was researching. I went through a lot of gymnastics, I was embarrassingly obnoxious, and I even impersonated a doctor to get an appointment with him. In fact, when the doctor met me, he said, "Who in the hell do you think you are?"*

Nevertheless, the doctor took Michelle as his patient, and she's doing well today.

This doesn't mean that cold calling won't work. Several interviewees described getting accepted by outstanding hospitals and surgeons that way. As mentioned earlier, **James' wife** successfully used faxed letters to seek medical consults when James was diagnosed with incurable multiple myeloma. Similarly, **Abby's sister** made a cold call to the Dana-Farber Cancer Institute, a prestigious comprehensive cancer treatment and research center in Boston, and got Abby accepted within two days.

While there's no one *right* way, it's certainly easier if you can network your way to a doctor; but if you must go at it cold, do so with confidence and persistence. The bottom line is: Do whatever is necessary to get the best medical team.

## Second Opinions

In some situations, it's worth the extra time to seek a second opinion while in others, any delay may jeopardize a patient's survival. A second opinion can give you additional information to validate the cancer diagnosis, provide further details, suggest a different course of treatment, or even determine that the cancer is a different type or stage. Such information can be confusing, but it will be less so if you coordinate through the doctor who provided the initial diagnosis. You may also want to check with your patient's health insurance plan to find out whether a second opinion is either required or covered.

Most doctors will fully support your desire for a second opinion and will refer you to an appropriate resource. Any physician who is reluctant to have you seek a second opinion is sending you a veiled message that he insists on being right and isn't willing to partner with you or with other physicians in planning your patient's care. Take the message and seek out a physician who is more willing to be responsive to your requests.

A second opinion is most useful in the following kinds of situations:[16]

- ஒ If the patient has been told that standard treatments are not working any longer and that no further treatment will be beneficial. There's nothing to lose in seeking a second opinion.

- ஒ If there is something "borderline" about the case (might or might not be operable, might or might not warrant adjuvant chemotherapy, and so on). In this case a second opinion might reveal some facts that move the case off of the fence, in one direction or the other.

- ஒ If you live in a rural area and want confirmation from an urban cancer center that your case can be handled locally without increasing the risks.

- ஒ If your patient has a rare cancer or a tumor that is in a particularly challenging location.

- ஒ If the diagnostic process hasn't found the primary site of the cancer. Cancer that spreads (metastasizes) will be the same cell type as the original cancer. It is important to know whether the cancer in question is a metastasis of another cancer or a totally new one, so a consult for a second opinion might be able to make that determination.

- ஒ If your doctor wants the patient to participate in his own clinical trial. In this situation, a second opinion could help ensure that your doctor doesn't let his self-interest guide his recommendation that you participate.

_____

16 *www.cancer.net*

To be most useful, a second opinion should be provided by an expert who practices independently of the diagnosing doctor. That way you'll get a totally fresh look. There are two types of doctors who may be involved in giving second opinions:

- Pathologist: A doctor who interprets your patient's biopsy or other laboratory results. If you have any question about the accuracy of the initial interpretation or if treatment options vary widely based on small variables in the pathology report, it may be worthwhile to consult with another pathologist.

- Oncologist or surgeon: A doctor who recommends the initial course of treatment, depending on which is the ideal first step.

Some cancer centers have a "tumor board," a multidisciplinary conference of doctors from different kinds of specialties. Such a resource can be very helpful if your doctor has any hesitation about the diagnosis or if you find yourself in a borderline situation of any kind. A tumor board can be accessed through your physician.

If you do decide to get a second opinion, obtain a copy of the patient's medical records, results from all scans, X-rays, and laboratory tests, and the pathology report. You must also obtain the cell slides from the laboratory where the original cells were examined. If the slides are being sent to another institution through the original doctor's office or the lab that did the tests, your patient may need to sign a release that will authorize them to be shared. If the second opinion is in your local area, you can obtain the slides in person and hand-carry them to the receiving institution.

There are two impartial resources that can help you find second opinion services:

- The R. A. Bloch Cancer Foundation *(www.blochcancer.org)* (800-433-0464). This foundation posts a list of "multidisciplinary" second opinion centers, listed by state.

- The National Institutes of Health (NIH) Clinical Center in Bethesda, MD *(www.cancer.gov/cancertopics)*, is the NIH

research hospital. Several NCI branches accessible there provide second opinion services.

You can also contact any major cancer center that is associated with a medical school or has its own research center.

Not every second opinion produces a significant change in direction
or intensity of treatment. In fact, many of the interviewees—like **Mike's
wife**—described getting second opinions that corroborated the original diagnosis and course of recommended treatment:

> *The messages from the doctors were negative from the be-
> ginning, from the diagnosis. We saw a second surgeon still
> hoping for surgery. This visit confirmed the first news. Mike
> asked this doctor for his advice and the doctor said, "Do
> nothing or give it hell." The morbidity of the disease was
> stunning to us. The prognosis for pancreatic cancer was four
> to six weeks. Mike lived 27 months.*

Mike and his wife didn't get a different opinion about the survivability
of his cancer, but the encouragement he did receive allowed him to fight
hard and far outlive his original prognosis.

## Switching Physicians or Hospitals

Some physicians exhibit such callous bedside manner or demonstrate such
an unwillingness to listen to your and your patient's concerns that you might
wonder how they can stay in business at all. Remember that only one quarter
of the nation's hospitals are certified by the Commission on Cancer, and even
fewer receive NCI cancer center or comprehensive cancer center certification. So just because you're in a hospital, you're not necessarily in the *right*
hospital. Some negative situations can be salvaged, especially if you're willing to meet the doctor halfway in improving the relationship and "fit." Others cannot, especially if your trust in your physician's judgment or reliability
or in the hospital's quality of care has been undermined.

Interviewees who had negative experiences were believers in being advocates for their loved ones. They agreed that no caregiver should tolerate

mishandling of a patient by any medical professional or institution or accept being treated as just a numbered clinical case. There's no excuse for bad manners on the part of any member of the medical team, and there's nothing wrong with following your instincts and pressing for appropriate and compassionate care.

Above all, caregivers say to trust your gut. If something feels wrong, it probably is. Take action before you have to get angry to get the needed care. Anger has no place in the cancer journey. In the end, it's your patient's life, so you and the patient should be in the driver's seat throughout the process.

While being diagnosed with stage III-C ovarian cancer, Abby experienced an extreme case of poor bedside manner by her prospective surgeon. **Abby's sister** relates how she and Abby immediately took charge of her health care situation:

> It was hard to change hospitals, but my gut feel was that the regional hospital's surgeon gave Abby an exam that was cruel and unnecessarily painful. She gave us a death sentence that we refused to accept. We wanted a doctor who would do more than postpone death and would give Abby a better quality of life. We didn't know what the research hospital in the city would say, but if you don't try, the answer is automatically no.

As the patient, **Abby** led the charge:

> Life is full of tough decisions. My gut feel about the surgeon was that to stay with that doctor would have been worse than doing nothing. It's not whether you live or die, but your quality of life that matters, and I didn't believe she could give me that. My gut feel was that I wasn't taking a big chance in the delay, even though I knew it was an aggressive cancer and getting worse.

In the end, the decision to go to a more specialized research hospital not only led to a different diagnosis—a less severe stage of her cancer— but required considerably less complex surgery than the local surgeon had planned and allowed for a faster recovery process. Despite having to travel farther from home, the sisters found that their medical team returned calls within 15 minutes. So far the outcome has been positive, and both of them are now optimistic.

If you do change physicians and/or hospitals, be prepared to take the initiative in getting your patient's files and records transferred (with authorization through your patient's signature or with yours if you hold a current medical power of attorney or health care proxy).[17] Also be prepared to share with the new team a detailed listing of all of your patient's medications, together with frequency and dosages, as well as key dates of various tests, scans, surgeries, radiation, chemotherapy, and so on from your patient's past treatment.

As a caregiver you should never feel hesitant to seek out another physician if you feel that the chemistry isn't right. The only cost to you is time and perhaps a duplicate consultation fee. The more comfortable you are with the "fit" that you and your patient have with your medical team leader, the more effective a caregiver you'll be, and the better the treatment your patient will get. In many cases, it's about trusting your gut instinct. It can't be said too often that if your gut tells you something is wrong, it's sending a message to your brain to listen!

---

17 A medical power of attorney is an instrument (or document) that allows a patient to appoint an agent (or proxy) to make health care decisions in the event that the patient is incapable of making such decisions (see Chapter Twelve, p. 198).

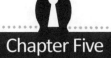

# Chapter Five

# Making Treatment Decisions

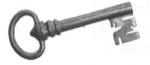

When preparing for your patient's cancer treatment, be prepared to ask more questions and to make more decisions. Cancer is a complex disease that may require multiple techniques either sequentially or simultaneously for its removal or control. You may also have access to treatment activities that are targeted to improve patient comfort or quality of life rather than removing or controlling the cancer itself. Treatment choices are generally framed against data that show how well certain treatments work against particular cancers.

By becoming familiar with the broad categories of treatments that might be offered to your patient, you'll be able to ask better questions and make better choices. Your choices are critical because certain treatment regimens (like radiation) cannot be repeated in the same location, and others represent either/or choices from the available options. Each treatment option also carries with it distinctive benefits, risks, and side effects which you'll want to understand in advance.

This chapter addresses six important topics that need to be understood as you make your choices:

**Standard-of-Care Protocols**

**Complementary Therapies**

**Clinical Trials**

**Genetic Testing**

**Alternative Therapies**

**Palliative Care**

## Standard-of-Care Protocols

The concept of standard of care (sometimes also called "best practice" or "the gold standard") refers to diagnostic and treatment protocols that have been proven empirically (over time and from large numbers of patient histories) to be the most successful for a particular type of cancer. For example, the standard of care for colon cancer screening is colonoscopy. There are other techniques—like virtual colonoscopy and CT colonography—which may be useful for people with average risk profiles, but colonoscopy has a better track record because it both finds polyps of any size and provides easy access for a surgeon to remove them during the same procedure. Other procedures may not give visibility to smaller polyps; if polyps are found, the patient would have to have a subsequent colonoscopy procedure for their removal and biopsy (requiring the patient to go through another bowel preparation process).

Many established treatment protocols involve some combination of distinctly different activities such as:

๛ Surgery (to remove a solid tumor or mass).

๛ Chemotherapy (to permeate the patient's entire body with a drug—by injection, infusion, or pill—to kill cancer cells that may be circulating in the blood or lymphatic system).

๛ Radiation (to shrink tumors and kill cancer cells in a specific location, thereby blocking disease spread or recurrence).

Generally the side effects and risks of these protocols are known and can be mitigated through supplemental medications that have proven to make patients more comfortable during treatment.

Standard-of-care procedures are delivered by licensed medical professionals and are supported by a combination of positive survival statistics and positive quality of life experiences for the majority of patients who receive them. One important resource for learning about these is the National Comprehensive Cancer Network (NCCN), a non-profit alliance of 26 leading cancer centers. Its mission is to improve the quality, effectiveness, and efficiency of oncology practice and to develop practice guidelines for use by patients, clinicians, and other decision-makers who influence cancer care delivery.

Based on research and analysis of its own experience serving more than 160,000 new patients each year, NCCN initiatives are designed to emphasize the importance of multidisciplinary services and the integration of patient care, research, and education. NCCN convenes panels of leading experts from around the country to identify the most effective treatments for various kinds of cancers. The goal for these panels is to identify best practices from across large patient populations and to translate complex clinical information into a consumer-friendly format. Guidelines for both physicians and patients are then disseminated for each cancer in both printed and electronic formats (including mobile applications).

Free patient guidelines for best practice treatments and options are available at the NCCN website *www.nccn.com*. Additional insights for caregivers are provided there, which represents an easy means of connecting with other Internet caregiver resources. NCCN can be reached by phone at 215-690-0300.

## Complementary Therapies

As they work through standard-of-care treatments, some patients turn to other kinds of therapies to improve their physical comfort. The most legitimate are known as complementary (also called integrative) therapies—non-medical approaches that can be used *in tandem with* traditional Western medical techniques. Complementary therapies may include acupuncture; dietary supplements (vitamins, probiotics, and so on); mind-body techniques like meditation, yoga, and guided imagery; massage; spinal manipulation; herbal or dietary treatment systems; and movement therapies like Pilates. They're primarily targeted toward improving the patient's quality of life.

Some hospitals make a wide variety of complementary services available. For instance, **Amelia's husband** suggested that:

> *If someone tells you that your treatment involves chemo and immediate symptom management, you need to think past the cancer. Talk with the dietician about food needs. Talk with palliative care about things to do to help get through the experience, like activities (art and music), writing to get your thoughts down on paper, Reiki massage, physical therapy, and so on.*

Still other hospitals incorporate the best of the complementary therapies into what they call integrated oncology practices. If you wish to find more information about complementary therapies, consult the National Center for Complementary and Alternative Medicine within the National Institutes of Health *(www.nccam.nih.gov)* or the Society for Integrative Oncology (SIO) *(www.integrativeonc.org)*, both of which focus on studying and facilitating cancer treatment and recovery through combinations of therapies.

The SIO seeks out information that will validate a treatment's claimed benefits and works to educate potential consumers. The SIO website also lists some of the well-established integrated oncology practices that research the efficacy of complementary therapies and advocate evidence-based therapies to improve quality of life for cancer patients. Such well-established practices include Mayo Clinic in Rochester, MN; the MD Anderson Cancer Center in Houston, TX; Memorial Sloan-Kettering Cancer Center in New York City; and the Zakim Center for Integrative Therapies at Dana-Farber Cancer Institute in Boston, MA.

## Clinical Trials

Standard-of-care therapies don't always produce the needed results for every patient. Clinical trials are often appropriate in such cases. According to the National Cancer Institute, a clinical trial is a study performed toward the end of a lengthy cancer research process. It involves administering a pre-determined drug regimen to cancer patients "to find out whether promising approaches to cancer prevention, diagnosis, and treatment are safe and effective."[18]

In cancer research today, each new discovery triggers more inquiries, all aimed toward finding new treatments. Genomic and microbiology researchers are seeking new means of attacking previously drug-resistant cancers. Others are looking at the potential for repurposing proven treatments for one cancer against others that have similar genetic profiles. Investigators are even exploring ways of using the body's immune system to fight a variety of caners. This means that the number of open clinical trials will be expanding but that the population sought for each will be tightly targeted.

Clinical trials may be conducted by a product manufacturer under the direction of the Food and Drug Administration. Pharmaceutical companies test new treatments, approaches to prevention, screening techniques, and the impact of treatments on patients' quality of life. Trials consist of four phases:

- ❧ Phase I asks "Is it safe?" Trials are conducted with animals and then with people to determine how a drug should best be delivered (by mouth, injection into the blood, injection into a muscle, and so on) and the safety and biological effects of alternative dosages.

- ❧ Phase II asks, "Does it work?," by continuing to test safety and effectiveness against particular types of cancer.

- ❧ Phase III asks, "Does it work better?," by comparing the new treatment to standard protocols, often with participants assigned at random to receive either the standard or the new drug.

---

18 Go to *www.cancer.gov* and search for "clinical trials."

✍ Phase IV, the final stage before a therapy is offered commer-
cially, asks, "Does it represent an improvement over existing treatments?" This phase evaluates the side effects, risks,
and benefits of the drug over a longer time period in a larger
number of people.[19] The goal of every clinical trial is to find
treatment protocols that produce significantly better outcomes
as measured in statistical terms.

For some caregivers, a clinical trial can produce a miracle, but for others
it may represent a promise pursued but not realized. The decision to participate in a clinical trial should not be taken lightly, because for many cancer
patients, the decision about whether to participate in a particular clinical
trial means choosing a path that will preclude other choices at a later date.

**Carole's husband** explained the clinical trials process from the caregiver's viewpoint:

> At the end of the day, you are presented with a Chinese menu
> saying, "OK, we have this study, this regimen, this treatment."
> The problem is that once you start making choices, you have
> closed off some other options. If you took W, you are auto-
> matically ineligible to take X, Y, or Z. Honestly, it's like play-
> ing Russian roulette, or the soup du jour. What's available
> today? These are your choices. The ultimate efficacy of any
> one protocol can't be known when you're making the choice
> of whether to participate.

For some patients, like James, various clinical trials have sustained his
life for many years and have beaten his cancer into a controllable state. For
others, like Mike S, they postponed his death for two years but didn't produce a cure. Still others found that a clinical trial didn't change the course
of the disease but may have added to researchers' understanding of certain cancers so that future patients will benefit. In short, clinical trials are

---

19  See the NIH website on clinical trials for a more detailed explanation of the
various stages of clinical trials and the pros and cons of participating
(*www.clinicaltrials.gov*).

research in motion; their pros and cons, their potential impacts, and the trade-offs they pose should be evaluated with care.

When it comes to a clinical trial, usually your oncologist will research and offer the appropriate clinical trial. Physicians who practice at research hospitals and major cancer centers tend to be knowledgeable about what's emerging in the world of clinical trials, so they represent the fastest route to learning whether such a trial is likely to help your patient.

Nevertheless, many caregivers feel an urgency to seek out a trial on their own. If you are inclined to do so, you need to work in conjunction with your physician. For more information, try searching at *www.clinicaltrials. gov* or go to the website for the American Cancer Society's Clinical Trials Matching Service at *www.cancer.org/treatment* and use the search function. You may need to partner with your physician in this process because the application forms require specific technical information (for example, cell type) from lab tests that will require access to the diagnostic details and ongoing medical monitoring of the patient's condition.

If and when you are considering clinical trial options, be sure to get answers to questions like:

- ❧ What's the trial's goal? Is it intended to cure the cancer (drive it into remission), stabilize the cancer, or simply improve the patient's quality of life?

- ❧ What are the probabilities of achieving that outcome or even better as compared with standard treatment? What exactly is the difference between the trial and that standard, and how does selection for the trial medication or procedure affect the probabilities of a successful outcome?

- ❧ How long will it take under the trial before we'll know whether it's working? How will you know?

- ❧ Can the trial be administered locally or at your current hospital of choice?

❧ How does participation open up or close off other treatment options if the trial isn't successful for your patient?

❧ How will the quality of your patient's life differ between standard treatment and the clinical trial protocol? Will side effects be predictable? Will they be better or worse than those in standard treatment?

These questions are essential not only to ensure that you make a good choice, but also to manage your expectations and those of your patient.

## Genetic Testing

Genetic testing was mentioned by only three caregivers. Yet the radical differences in the reason why each chose to pursue testing, and the impact for each, reflects the range in actual and potential uses for DNA technology. It's important for family caregivers to understand how such genetic tests might affect the patient's relatives.

Genetic testing is becoming a powerful tool in the cancer fighter's arsenal. The National Cancer Institute (within the U.S. National Institutes of Health) claims that genetic information is now helping scientists and physicians to:

❧ Identify those at risk from certain kinds of cancers (primarily breast, ovarian, colorectal, and thyroid), especially when a hereditary pattern might be suspected.

❧ Understand cell biology and the nature of cell mutations. (The word "mutation" is used by NCI to refer to a change or disruption in the normal DNA sequence of a particular gene, which changes its behavior and may cause cancer.)

❧ Characterize the extent and seriousness of certain malignancies.

❧ Define what treatment regimen is most appropriate to the "molecular fingerprint" of a given person's disease.

❧ Discover new therapies to treat certain forms of cancer.[20]

---

20 *www.cancer.gov/cancertopics.*

Interviewees offered three examples of potential positive impacts of exploring genetic testing. The first saved a life, the second found undiagnosed cancers among other family members, and the third helped refine a diagnosis.

**Tahira's mother** explained that a genetic test may have saved her life. Tahira was 33 when she was diagnosed with breast cancer. Because her family history included several generations of breast cancer on her mother's side of the family, she had had a baseline mammogram beginning at age 29. At age 32 her mammogram was clear, but six months later she felt a lump in her breast:

> *The mammogram showed a five-centimeter mass, and by the time an ultrasound was done, they said it had grown to six or seven centimeters. The surgeon described it as having gone from a popcorn-sized grain to fully popped popcorn in size over a short period. He suggested a mastectomy and reconstruction because the tumor was too large to get out through only one angle, and he wanted both to be safe and to avoid multiple cuts that would be unsightly. Five days after surgery and reconstruction, when the pathology report came out, the doctor said, "You're done, and you'll be good."*
>
> *Then, another five days later, we got a call asking all three of us to come in to talk with another pathologist. She had heard about Tahira's case, and because Tahira was so young, she wanted to look at the slides with regard to the BRCA gene.[21] When she did, she saw a strong presence of HER2/neu visible on the slide. HER2 is an enzyme directing cells to grow, and because there was no way to know where those cells had gone to grow, she felt Tahira should have a full course of chemotherapy. This came to us out of the blue. We're grateful that this pathologist was interested enough to take another look.*

---

21  In normal cells, two genes (known as BRCA1 and BRCA2) help prevent uncontrolled cell growth. Mutation of these genes has been linked to the development of hereditary breast and ovarian cancer. Go to *http://www.cancer.gov* and search for BRCA.

Despite Tahira's family history of breast cancer for her mother, grand-mother, and grandmother's sister, her surgeon hadn't ordered a genetic test, and the first pathologist didn't look for the BRCA genetic markers on the surgical tissue sample. Fortunately, a potential subsequent medical crisis was averted by a curious and patient-oriented pathologist who hadn't even been assigned to her case.

Michael S was 17 when he was diagnosed with his medullary thyroid carcinoma (MTC). Only 4% of all cancer patients have thyroid cancer, and only 1% of those have MTC. **Michael S's father** was concerned:

> *Michael's cancer was so rare that the average patient is a 54-year-old woman. The doctor had never seen it in a 17-year-old male, so he believed it might be genetic. The only lab that could do the test was the Mayo Clinic, so that meant a four- to six-week wait between doing the test and getting results.*
>
> *The immediate family was tested, and my wife learned that she had the gene. My wife's family got tested, and we found that her mother and one of her sisters also had it; one sister didn't. All three of them had the gene and were showing signs of cancer, but Michael's was more advanced. None of them needed radiation, but all of them had the surgery.*
>
> *The testing also identified that my wife also had an adrenal tumor known as Pheo [pheochromocytoma]. If they had not operated on the adrenal glands first to remove that tumor, the thyroid cancer surgery would have killed her because it would have caused her heart to beat too fast, in overdrive. Each of the members of her family presented differently. We went the whole way as soon as the diagnosis came in.*

Michael S's thyroid cancer—which is still proving to be an ongoing challenge for Michael—and the subsequent genetic test proved to be a life-saver for other members of his family.

As **Brian's wife** recounts, a genetic test helped identify the exact nature of her husband's cancer so that he could be given the proper treatment:

> *They did genetic testing with both of the biopsies (the origi-nal one done by the hematologist and a second biopsy per-formed by another hospital). They found out exactly what they were dealing with. It took us from the worst category to the intermediate category.*
>
> *That made all the difference, to have hope. Now they're keep-ing him in remission, but he's not yet healthy. Leukemia re-missions always fail; it's always a matter of time, so he'll need a bone marrow transplant in the future. That's his best shot for a cure, but they've made great progress with his treatment.*

If you are interested in learning more about genetic testing, there are several useful Internet websites:

- *www.ghr.nlm.nih.gov*, the website for the Genetics Home Ref-erence of the National Library of Medicine, within the NCI, allows you to get live help on genetic questions about cancer and to get information on what types of cancer have suspected hereditary links.

- *www.facingourrisk.org*. This is the website of Force (Facing Our Risk of Cancer Empowered), a nonprofit organization focused on providing support, education, advocacy, aware-ness, and research in the area of hereditary breast and ovar-ian cancer.

- The Genetic and Rare Diseases Information Center (GARD) of the National Institutes of Health can be reached at *www.rarediseases.info.nih.gov*. It was established by the National Human Genome Research Institute and the Office of Rare Diseases Research.

Current breakthrough research projects suggest that in the future, physicians will draw increasingly on genetic testing to identify which treatments are likely to produce the best outcomes for each patient and even to develop personalized treatment protocols. One example of this work that has breathtaking implications is the Circulating Tumor Cell Center at Massachusetts General Hospital. More information is available at *www.massgeneral.org/research.*

## Alternative Therapies

There are other treatments available to cancer patients that are sometimes touted by their practitioners to be used *instead of* traditional therapies. They are usually referred to as alternative therapies. Such treatments may look attractive to patients for whom traditional approaches are no longer working or offer little promise of survival. Many of them are controversial, and there is little empirical evidence that they produce the desired outcomes. Most of them come with expensive, supposedly proprietary products claiming near-miracle cures, together with a series of costly in-office protocols for applying or infusing those products.

Responsible oncologists practice evidence-based medicine and prescribe treatment protocols that are supported by empirical data showing their effectiveness. As a result, they may express alarm when a patient suggests replacing traditional therapy with an alternative, or engaging in a therapy that will conflict with the clinical treatments that are underway. Many oncologists also consider alternative treatments as nothing more than a money pit constructed by "snake oil salesmen," charlatans who fleece patients and prey on their desperation. **Bruce MacDonald** explains that:

> *There's absolutely a bias in a research cancer hospital toward treatments and approaches that have been approved with empirical evidence to support their efficacy. Therefore newer treatments, somewhat far-out treatments, or alternative treatments are not exactly frowned upon, but they're not presented as options because some oncologists see them as voodoo medicine.*

Ned, a patient for metastasized prostate cancer, is an example of a patient who mistakenly relied on alternative medicine. He ended up caught between his adult children, who were pushing him toward alternative treatments, and his wife, who believed that the children were demonizing Western medicine and pressuring him to use unproven treatments. **Ned's wife** says that as a result of their pressure, he became indecisive, which set back his progress within standard-of-care treatments:

> *There weren't any empirical data available about the impact or success rate of the alternative treatments that the kids were pushing on him. Also, these treatments (one of which cost $5,000 per week) weren't covered by insurance.*
>
> *Close to eight months later, Ned wasn't making a decision about which therapy to follow—starting chemo at the cancer center or pursuing an alternative treatment. His oncologist forced the issue by saying, "You can have two different side effects from delay. One is the side effects of chemo, which I can get you through, and the other is the side effects of cancer, which you won't live through. The last scan we did showed only a couple of places where cancer was in your bones. Now I can stick a needle into any bone in your body and find cancer cells. My prediction is that if you don't start something very quickly, you'll be dead within six to eight months."*

Ned continued stubbornly resisting chemotherapy and pursued the costly alternative treatments his children had suggested. After he had several emergency hospitalizations in rapid succession, **Ned's wife** reported that he finally

> *didn't want to go for the alternative treatments anymore. He started on a low-dose chemo at his original cancer center. After three treatments, one a week, for symptom treatment only, he had gained 10 pounds, his PSA was a quarter of what it was when he started, and he played his first set of doubles tennis that weekend. It was like a miracle.*

Unfortunately, Ned resumed chemotherapy too late and died several months later.

Other caregivers and their patients rejected such treatments. Even though the initial diagnosis for Patti indicated that she was terminal, **Patti's daughter** was unequivocal about her disdain for alternative treatments:

> *Don't believe everything you read. There are lots of quack cures you should ignore. It's easy to believe they can help when you want them to.*

Your patient's oncologist can help determine whether the alternative remedies you are considering will interact negatively with any of your ongoing standard treatments and physical conditions. If there is no conflict, the physician may be able to provide you with a referral to a qualified practitioner. Even so, it is important to scrutinize that practitioner in the same way you would scrutinize your oncology team. In addition, be sure to find out:

- ~ Does the alternative treatment practitioner also sell products? (If so, this can suggest that the practice is intended as a "feeder" into product sales and may make the individual's professionalism suspect.)

- ~ Are any aspects of the treatment or products used certified by the U.S. Food and Drug Administration?

- ~ What will be the cost of treatment? Is the cost covered by the patient's insurance? (This is important. Remember Ned's $5,000 per week out-of-pocket cost.)

It is understandable that when things look hopeless, some patients and their caregivers will clutch at any straws. The patient may feel desperate, but it's important for the caregiver to serve as the voice of reason. The message from most of the interviewees about alternative treatments is to do your homework and ask for empirical evidence that they work. If there isn't any, and especially if the alternative provider is selling costly nutritional supplements that are masquerading as chemotherapy, the treatments may only yield false hope and big expenses.

## Palliative Care

Palliative care focuses on helping the patient improve his quality of life by providing relief from pain and other discomforts that may accompany the disease or its treatment. It is often provided in the hospital and may be covered by medical insurance. Palliative care has become an accepted specialty that includes doctors, nurses, social workers, counselors, chaplains, massage therapists, nutritionists, pharmacists and a variety of providers of complementary services.

Some cancer patients are referred to palliative care soon after diagnosis to help them cope with physical, emotional, and/or psychological discomfort, which may include symptoms such as pain, nausea, breathing problems, muscle spasms, fatigue, constipation or diarrhea, sleeping difficulties, eating difficulties, or anxiety. Palliative care professionals can coordinate with the primary cancer care team to ensure that your patient understands available treatment choices and the implications of each.

Dr. Jennifer Temel of Massachusetts General Hospital conducted a clinical trial on palliative care in treating stage IV non-small cell lung cancer patients by incorporating early palliative care into their standard treatment plans. Results were sufficiently striking—in improving quality of life, reducing rates of depression, diminishing the need for aggressive care at the end of life, and increasing median survival period—that they are being called "paradigm shifting." For more information, see *www.asco.org* and insert "Jennifer Temel" in the search engine.

You can get more information about palliative care services either from your patient's oncologist or from *www.getpalliativecare.org*. In addition, pain control is becoming a medical sub-specialty of its own. Ask your patient's oncologist for suggestions or visit one of the following links and search "pain control":

- ≈ *www.cancer.gov/cancertopics*
- ≈ *www.cancer.org/Treatment*

Not all oncologists are yet fully knowledgeable about palliative care techniques, so don't relent in pressing for nausea, pain, and anxiety relief.

Palliative care is also an important feature of hospice services, which are addressed in Chapter Twelve, below.

Becoming familiar with the key terms the medical team will use in discussing treatment options is an important foundation for you as you move into the most critical phase of your cancer caregiving. With this understanding, you'll be well-equipped to serve as a proactive liaison between your patient and the medical practitioners you've chosen to spearhead his care. The next chapter will help you get your head around the range of activities that you're likely to encounter.

# Chapter Six

# Getting Inside the Caregiver Role

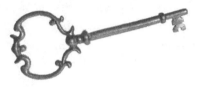

Caregiving means playing many different roles, including coach, sounding board, mediator, information gatherer, or a shoulder to cry on. Few cancers can be treated with a single silver bullet, and everything we normally count on is likely to be in flux as the patient goes through treatment. While you may be called on to perform many tasks, your overriding responsibility is to become your patient's advocate throughout the experience, no matter what challenges arise.

**Bruce MacDonald** put the role in perspective based on his years of experience working with cancer patients and their caregivers:

> *If you define advocacy as an expression of love, my caregiver is somebody who's desperately trying to avoid losing me. I think that for most patients that I've known who had a very aggressive advocate caregiver, it's enormously comforting to know that there is somebody other than myself who is watching out for me, and whose brain right now is more adept at formulating conversations and ideas and at researching, because I'm sick or exhausted or scared.*

For some patients, like **Judy M**, what the caregiver does isn't the most important factor:

*My husband's greatest support was accepting me for who
I was. I had my head shaved; I was throwing up, sleeping
through weekends, and not feeling that great when I was
awake. I had seen my mother's frustration when my father's
health declined, and I wondered if it would happen to us. But
he was there. It wasn't what he did, but that he was there.*

**Paul's wife** learned a similar lesson when she tried to help her
husband in her own way, rather than his:

*At first, as caregiver, I felt the need to take care of Paul. He
was really scared and both withdrawn and depressed. He
was angry because I wanted to do things to help him and
tried to be a cheerleader. He got upset and said he needed to
feel the feelings he was having, and he resented my trying to
cheer him up.*

Because each caregiver has to forge his own unique partnership with
his patient, this chapter addresses eight aspects of the caregiving process
and experience:

> **Managing HIPPA Issues**
>
> **Learning to Give Up Control**
>
> **Taking an Active Role at Medical Appointments**
>
> **Advocating Effectively for Your Patient**
>
> **Disagreeing Without Being Disagreeable**
>
> **Building Relationships with Professional Caregivers**
>
> **Letting the Patient Call the Shots**
>
> **Keeping Hope Alive**

## Managing HIPPA Issues

You can't be an effective advocate without access to the patient's medical information. The passage of the Health Insurance Portability and
Accountability Act of 1996 (HIPAA) requires medical providers to ensure
the privacy of each patient's medical records.

Your patient's medical data are his own unless he signs a form giving you access. If the patient is not conscious or cannot give permission, health care providers may discuss the health information with the designated caregiver if they believe it is in the patient's better interests. Even if the patient has signed a HIPAA form for a particular medical office, the information may only be shared as it relates to the current medical matter, unless the patient has authorized broader sharing in advance with that provider.

In summary, the HIPAA form that he will sign specifies the organization that can release the data to you. Each health care provider may have different rules for verifying who may access the medical records, so a separate form needs to be completed for each medical provider who is in a different business organization. You will need that authorization for every organization that deals with your patient.

Even if your patient has signed a medical power of attorney or health care proxy (as discussed in Chapter Twelve), you will probably need to have him sign HIPAA forms as well because those documents only become active if the patient has lost the capacity to make or communicate medical decisions. When you create your medical power of attorney, you may want to try including a blanket authorization for you to have access to all medical records, but there is no guarantee that every medical provider will agree to honor it while the patient is fully alert and in competent condition. As a result, you would do well to complete the HIPAA privacy release forms,[22] leaving the medical provider blank, and then make multiple copies so you can fill in the specific provider's identity when necessary.

## Learning to Give Up Control

In the normal routines of life, most of us want to believe that there are some things we can control, that events aren't happening at random or in reaction to forces beyond our understanding. A cancer diagnosis tests that conviction to the limits, even for people who don't consider themselves "control freaks."

---

22  A HIPAA privacy release form can be found by searching at
    *http://www.caring.com*. Use the search engine to find "HIPPA release form."

Everyone copes with the loss of control in different ways. One husband of a terminal cancer patient made a serious pass at his wife's best friend, who also served as her caregiver. It caused awkwardness, making the friend back away from any situation where he might be present. Another caregiver, the wife of a seriously ill cancer patient, went into therapy because her fear of being abandoned had led to her developing a crush on another man. As she described the problem:

> It was a coping mechanism, finding a back-up in case my husband died, so I wouldn't be alone. The other guy and I would hang out frequently, but he backed out of it and walked away, which was a good thing. The life and death stuff is really terrifying.

Fortunately, her husband recovered, and they are doing well today.

One of the most important issues for cancer caregivers is to acknowledge the things that are beyond their control. These things are what they are, so don't waste time and energy on them. For those who are used to living a fairly structured life, giving up control may make the adjustment to cancer caregiving especially unsettling.

**Jen P's husband** works in the financial services industry and relies on highly structured data for use in decision-making. When Jen's cancer hit, his personality made things difficult for him:

> I'm an organization freak. I've got to have things just so. I had a notebook, tabs, phone numbers. When I realized I didn't have control, it wasn't good. Plenty of nights I'd run longer because I was so frustrated. You have to play the cards you were dealt.

Having already lost two siblings to cancer, **Michelle's husband** admits he also has control issues and that he is persistent almost to a fault:

> I'm a control guy. I don't lose. I didn't balance things very well. I was going to tough it out, work harder, and do whatever it took. I did just that even more after my sister's death. The cancer patient feels a loss of control and a loss of normal life. That's the greatest fear for caregivers. You can do things

*to improve the odds, to make treatments better, and to help people die better. But if you are looking at outcomes, you just don't have that control.*

**Jenn S's husband**, a biomedical project manager, applied his desire to maintain in control to all aspects of Jenn's care. He now realizes he should have allowed others to be more engaged so Jenn would have had a broader support network, and he would have had more help in caring for her:

*The thing I'd do differently if I had it to do again is give others more access to her. That's one of the hard things for me to do. I've got what could politely be called "control issues." The cancer made it worse.*

*Letting others care for her was hard. Even letting her brothers or mother or dad take care of her was hard for me. Sometimes individuals made poor choices and earned their way out of caregiving, but other times I've been too stubborn and controlling to let that happen. It was hard.*

His stubbornness had a positive side, however, when he refused to remove Jenn from life support:

*I wasn't particularly popular with members of our families because I wanted to keep Jenn on life support. They said I was selfish. I faced a lot of criticism for being willing to put her through that in the hopes she'd come out on the other side. They judged me. When she lived, I didn't get any apologies from them on the other side.*

Many caregivers recommend that you look for areas in your life that you *can* control and identify how you may approach them differently in order to take advantage of the freedom that remains. For example, **Mindy's husband** found that their oncologist's approach to help Mindy get through a specific treatment plan over a defined period of time was accompanied by beneficial counseling about their perceived loss of control:

*He made it clear that we could still control how we took care of the kids. He didn't tell us how to do it, but we had read*

*ACS books and talked to others who had had cancer. The best advice was to be honest but not necessarily detailed. You can't hide the side effects of chemo, or the fact that sometimes you'll cry in front of them, and they need to know why and that it's not only Dad who's a caregiver.*

Your patient may need help in dealing with his own control issues and will benefit from being able to take charge in some aspects of his life. **Mike S's wife** tried to identify ways her husband could reestablish control after the cancer diagnosis took it away:

*Mike wanted options. That was his way of exerting control, to have treatment choices. In fact, my "research" just helped us feel in control.*

For **Brian's wife**, the lack of control stimulated the fight for recovery:

*The risk factors for the leukemia are pretty vague, and not predictable. People who have them don't get it, and people who don't have them do get it. It's hard to adjust to. You want to feel you have some control and are doing the best you can until this happens, so it makes you angry. What do you do with the anger? You channel it into getting better.*

In summary, the caregivers' messages to you and your patient are to control what you can, acknowledge those factors that are beyond your power, and go with the flow as well as you can.

## Taking an Active Role at Medical Appointments

Cancer patients are awash in emotions—especially right after the diagnosis—and it may make it hard to hear and remember the details of what their physicians say to them. That's why many caregivers accompany their patients to every medical appointment and try to serve as their eyes and ears. It's not that caregivers don't also have those feelings, but they're better able to put them aside temporarily in the interests of helping the patient digest and evaluate what's happening in the moment.

As a nurse and a breast cancer survivor herself, **Tahira's mom** has a unique perspective:

> *I can tell you that medicine today is on a time clock, so doctors talk specifics of what they will do, but they don't get into perimeter stuff unless you ask. Patients have questions like: How long will I be out of work after surgery? Can I work during chemo? What can I do during radiation?*
>
> *The caregiver represents a second pair of ears. The caregiver helps them think how to plan out the next period of life financially, how to help both stay motivated during treatment, and how to handle changes in daily routines and schedules. The caregiver can help put plans in place so the patient doesn't have to worry.*

Some caregivers who know their own limitations will even enlist a third party to accompany them. **Carole's husband** explains how a third party became an important resource in their struggle with Carole's ovarian cancer:

> *There were times we brought a friend of Carole's, who was a nurse. I knew that I couldn't always be emotionally there. It's important at times to bring someone who's not as emotionally involved and who has enough medical knowledge to understand what's being said.*

There are specific ways caregivers can fulfill their roles as their patients' eyes and ears.

## Make Records of Information Conveyed by the Doctor

Keeping careful records is at the core of effective caregiving, and it begins at medical appointments. There's an enormous amount of information being exchanged, most of it in a foreign language I call "doctor-speak." If you're lucky, your physician and other medical professionals will translate doctor-speak into layman's English. If not, you'll want to make sure you keep track of the terms you need to research or learn more about. Keeping thorough notes while your patient is emotionally distracted by his cancer diagnosis will make it possible for you to go over the doctor's comments later, when he can absorb what the information means.

In the process, you may learn things about your patient that will surprise you and shape your caregiving role. That's what happened to **Tom's wife**, who after a 30-year marriage saw her husband in a new light after he was diagnosed with cancer:

> *Tom shuts down when he gets bad news, so my role as caregiver is to wake him up. You can actually see it on Tom's face; he just goes away. I only discovered this recently. The doctor will ask, "What do you think?," and Tom just sighs. I'd just be scribbling notes as fast as I could when we were with the doctor, and I wasn't looking at him for so long that I didn't realize what was happening. So now we drive home, and we talk, and then a few days later I'll call the doctor with his answer.*

Kathy is a serial caregiver—as **Jim's daughter, Artie's daughter-in-law**, and finally **Deb's sister**. She understands that different patients require different approaches, but she has also reached some general conclusions based on her experiences:

> *The patient only processes 0 to 50% of what he hears. There are new questions every week about what's been happening. You have to keep a notebook. Keep track of what's said at appointments. Make sure you write down the schedule and dosage of medications, and the possible side effects, and if you're getting medications prescribed by more than one doctor, check on interactions just in case the doctors didn't. Ensure that the doctors check the med list every single time, and keep it with you. My brother-in-law says they never told them that my sister's chemo would last six months, but it was definitely in the notebook.*

Add to this the fact that studies indicate that even at the best of times, most people can remember barely 25% of what they heard 24 hours earlier—we are much more visually oriented—and it becomes clear that taking good notes is one of the most essential activities a caregiver can perform.

For some, like **Mike S's wife**, using a small digital tape recorder can be easier than taking detailed notes. That strategy helped late one night when Mike misremembered a conversation with his oncologist about the prognosis for his pancreatic cancer:

> *The doctors were easy with my recording the visits, believing it helps impart accurate information. Sometimes I transcribed the conversations to help me organize my thoughts.*
>
> *At one visit, far along in the disease, we had been reviewing several options with Dr. C, and Mike said, "If I do nothing, how much time do I have?" Dr. C answered that it wouldn't be much time. Then the conversation continued, and we decided on one of the clinical trials as the next treatment.*
>
> *That night, I woke up to hear Mike crying. He whispered, "I only have a few weeks to live." I said, "Hold on just a minute." I was able to click on the tape recorder. We heard Mike ask, "If I do nothing...?" and then the rest of what Dr. C said about the next treatment.*

The doctor hadn't given up on Mike, and hearing him say that again helped soothe Mike's temporary feelings of desperation. If you do use the tape recording strategy, you'll want either to keep a log of how to access each conversation or to type them up for easy access later.

### Convey Patient Information To The Doctor

The flow of information between patient and doctor needs to be a two-way street. As the caregiver, you're more likely to be the objective party. You're not drugged, or in physical pain, or in a cancer-induced state of anxiety or distraction. That's why you need to be the one who keeps an eye on the kinds of symptoms that arise between medical visits. Even small things—like increasing thirst, a rash, sweats, or a new pain—can be important signals of how the treatments are working, and they need to be conveyed to the doctor.

Reporting such interim symptoms can usually wait until the next appointment. But if there are serious symptoms involving sustained vomiting or diarrhea that could leave your patient dehydrated, or if there's bleeding or difficulty breathing, you should call the physician or hospital immediately.

Caregivers say this is an important part of their jobs because their loved ones are sometimes oblivious to the little things or have difficulty differentiating between the good days and the not-so-good ones. For example:

> **René's wife** *There are times when the doctor will ask how are you doing. René will say, "I'm fine," and at the moment he is fine. I don't want to overstep, but there are things I know that are symptoms that the doctor needs to really know about. There's a discrepancy in communication between patients and doctors, and that's one of the reasons it's important to have an advocate for the patient and to have a doctor who asks more than yes/no questions.*

> **Mike S's wife** *Cancer patients worry that each symptom might signal new disease. During a course of chemo, Mike started to hiccup one evening. At first we laughed, then we became annoyed, and finally exhausted. It slowed down just enough for him to sleep. The next day I told the nurse practitioner, and she told us it is one of the side effects of chemo, an inflammation of the esophagus. She wrote out a prescription for medication to make the hiccups stop. We learned that the symptoms don't have to be a sign of disease progression; often they can be treated, and minimizing discomfort is an important part of treatment.*

You're not intruding if you track and report unexpected symptoms; in fact, you just may be providing an invaluable clue to doctors, not just helping to relieve unnecessary patient discomfort. **Richard's wife** had exactly that experience:

> *They told me that if he got a fever, I should call them. One night, when I touched Richard, he was wicked hot. I called and they told me to bring him to the emergency room. They*

*took one look and decided that they were going to keep him. Richard was really angry and said "I'm never coming here again." I had to come home for something the next day, and he called me and said, "If I hadn't gone to the hospital, I'd have been dead in six hours." It turns out that he had a blood infection that could have killed him.*

The advice from caregivers is to keep in touch with the medical team or the hospital if anything unexpected happens. It could mean the difference between life and death.

## Prepare Your Questions in Advance

From the moment the diagnosis is delivered, most cancer patients and their caregivers experience a flood of questions. **Mindy's husband** explains:

*My first thoughts were "where do we go from here?" I had lots of questions. How fast will it go? What do we do next? My brain was on overload with questions and scenarios. How do we do this? How do we tell the kids, who were 11, 9, and 3 at the time?*

Preparing questions in advance is a mechanism for bringing focus and structure to your thinking so your emotional reactions don't totally overwhelm your reasoning. Several caregivers advocated preparing questions in advance:

**Michelle's husband** *I brought typed questions with lots of space to write out the answers. It takes a load off the patient if the caregiver will do that.*

**Ellen's husband** *You've got to go armed with all the right questions and take careful notes.*

**Michael L's mother** *I had a notebook recording the protocols, side effects, and so on. It was my bible. I'd put my questions and their answers in it.*

Formulating your questions in advance will allow you to use your doctor's time most efficiently while ensuring that you raise all of your concerns and get the information you need. Part of this process is ensuring that you have the opportunity to reflect and come to grips with the truth so you can effectively manage your own expectations and those of your patient.

For many caregivers, asking questions of the doctor is essential for surviving the experience, both to help the patient and to maintain some sense of control over what's happening. It's hard to get the best out of your time together if you have to formulate your questions on the spot. Some of your questions may be triggered by the uncertainties of a challenging diagnosis. Specific questions about treatment options and their impacts are perfectly appropriate. They may arise in more casual conversation at home when you're not in the sometimes-anxious setting of the medical office.

## Advocating Effectively for Your Patient

The dictionary definition of an advocate is: "Somebody who acts or intercedes on behalf of another." Almost all of the caregivers interviewed for this book agreed that advocacy was their primary role. Some also saw themselves as their patient's protector from unnecessarily intrusive procedures or inexperienced hospital personnel. Others dealt with information gathering and decision-making support so their patient could focus on getting through treatment. Still others considered themselves buffers between the institution and the patient, committed to ensuring that his quality of life remained as good as possible, even in the hospital.

**Carl's wife**, who is a professional social worker by training, explained the need to take a consumer perspective:

> Be able to identify what you need or don't need. Professional people need to be able to give you what you need and not what they want to give you. You're a consumer, and their job should be to satisfy you.

As hard as you try, sometimes you may not get the answers you seek. When treatment options pose difficult choices, many doctors are reluctant to make a recommendation. In part, they want the patient to be the decision-maker in order to avoid feeling responsible if the results don't turn out to be positive. Sometimes they remain neutral when they truly do not know which option is best. **Ellen M's husband** suggested a strategy for getting a response if this kind of situation should arise:

> *Doctors try to de-personalize what they're doing, but when you ask them a certain question, it forces them to answer you in a very personal way. Don't be afraid to ask, "What if I were a really close family member? What would you recommend?" You'll get a more realistic appraisal from the physician.*

In the end, caregiving is about being an informed, engaged, and proactive advocate. If you don't get the clear answer you're seeking, try to ask the question in another way until you're satisfied. Then you may get a response you can interpret and understand, even if it's not as direct as you would have liked.

The role of advocate as a combination of support and protection is especially important if and when the patient is in the hospital because so many people beyond your primary cancer physician are in direct contact with him:

> **Didier's wife** *No one should have to go on the cancer journey alone. It could be your secretary, your business partner, your husband, your daughter—somebody should always be beside the patient.*

> **Mike S's wife** *I was in there like a crazy person. Sometimes, I'd even take my own breath away. If someone would come in to do a procedure, I'd ask how many of these have you done. If they weren't expert, I'd insist that a more senior fellow or the attending physician perform the procedure. Inexperience can mean that procedures take longer or might need to be repeated. Very ill patients need to be spared every possible discomfort.*

> **Trudy's domestic partner** *I've learned not to leave her side when she's in the hospital unless someone else is with*

*her. She has a phone and a pager for reaching me if I'm not there. Once, when she was in the hospital, we found out she was allergic to morphine but was OK with Fentanyl. It was put into her medical records. Only a few weeks later, when she was admitted for different surgeries, they were about to give her morphine, but I stopped them. It turns out that the doctor who wrote the morphine order hadn't read it on the record. I learned not to trust the medical system.*

Keeping a watchful eye on medical professionals is important because caring for a hospitalized patient involves so many different people, and not all of them read patient's records carefully. You also may need to bird-dog the medical records that follow your loved one through the various stages of his care. The health care system is filled with hand-offs from one medical professional to the next, creating plenty of opportunity for information to be lost, recorded incorrectly, or simply overlooked.

The bottom line on being an advocate is that if your gut tells you something isn't right, ask the professional caregivers to explain what they are doing and why, and to change it if necessary. If the answer doesn't satisfy you, ask to see the supervising nurse or doctor. It's perfectly acceptable to do so and to work your way up the chain of command because you're the stand-in for your patient. You are both consumers in the health care system, and have a right to receive clear, credible explanations and to correct any situation that may jeopardize the patient's physical or psychological well-being.

## Disagreeing Without Being Disagreeable

As an oncology social worker, **Bruce MacDonald** deals with sensitive caregiving situations every day and sometimes finds himself called in to help resolve disagreements among doctors, patients, and assertive caregivers:

*Sometimes physicians will bristle at that kind of caregiver, but so what. It's fairly rare, but sometimes you'll see a caregiver who's not only advocating—he's angry: Angry that this has happened, angry that there's no cure, or angry that it feels as though medical science is failing his loved one.*

> *That anger is at the cancer; it's anger at the situation. It's like striking your fist at the heavens, but sometimes it comes out personally at the medical team. Sometimes it's also anger that the caregiver or patient perceives that they were not really told all of the information that they feel they should have been told or wish they'd been told. That's legitimate righteous anger.*

> *Nevertheless, when doctors feel blamed or that someone's shaking a finger at them, they react. We're not all right out of our "Buddha" training discussions. It's in the heat of the moment. Doctors and nurses are all human.*

It's understandable that you might have difficulty managing your emotions if you believed your concerns weren't being heard or taken seriously by professional caregivers. Yet it's important to learn how to disagree with them in a respectful manner that conveys how you value their training even if you disagree with something that is happening at the moment.

Pushing back without anger is a challenge when you're so emotionally engaged in helping your patient through a difficult cancer experience, as **Jenn S's husband** learned:

> *As soon as you start yelling, people tune you out. I just tried very hard to be as calm and articulate as I could be and get my point across. If you do that enough, people have a certain level of respect for your credibility, so if you lose control of your emotions once, they won't hold it against you.*

In the end, disagreeing or challenging members of the medical team constructively means balancing your desire for action with your willingness to demonstrate respect and congeniality. If you are too "nice," you may back off too soon, but if you press too hard for action, you're likely to offend and generate counter-productive results. In the event that you feel too emotionally engaged to sustain a good balance, consider bringing in a more objective third party—a social worker or a friend or relative who has some medical, psychology or mediation training.

Above all, know to take a deep breath when you feel your emotions slipping out of control. If necessary, you might even want to ask that the particular procedure in question be postponed long enough to allow time for a calm, reasoned discussion with the responsible physician.

## Building Relationships with Professional Caregivers

For people who don't have a lot of history with hospitals and medical issues, it's sometimes hard to get used to the variety of treatment locales and personnel that will be involved in your patient's care. Because the patient may be moving in and out of a series of hospitals, chemotherapy infusion clinics, radiation centers, or doctors' offices, building good personal relationships with the people you have to deal with most frequently can pay invaluable dividends for both caregivers and patients, often in the form of more attentive and personalized treatment.

Although the two examples below both occurred with terminal patients, they are relevant to all patients:

> **Mike S's wife** *Early on, we were walking in the hospital, and Mike was saying hello to everyone he passed. I asked him why, and he said he knew he'd be spending a lot of time here, so he wanted to make some friends. Soon Mike knew little details about people he liked, such as the nurse who exercised regularly by doing belly dancing. That gave them something other than cancer to talk about. When he looked well, there were friends to celebrate, and if he were having a bad day, they'd say, "There's always tomorrow."*
>
> *He got to know one of the parking valets well. One day the valet opened the car door, looked at Mike, and burst into tears. "He's dying," he sobbed. It meant a lot to me that the valet, who had seen countless patients come and go, was brought to tears when Mike was dying. Now that I am left with only memories, I am grateful that Mike was cared for by people who genuinely cared about him.*
>
> **Joe's wife** *He always knew what was going on in these people's lives. If he asked them how they were, he really wanted*

*to know. When he was having chemo, he always brought the nurses a bouquet of flowers he'd grown.*

*After he decided he didn't want any more treatment, I can remember those nurses coming in at night and singing "Amazing Grace" to him. One night they put him in a lift and sat him in a tub to give him a bath. It took a cast of thousands, but they'll never know what that meant to him, because he was meticulous in his grooming.*

Both Mike and Joe taught personal caregivers important lessons about relationships. For some of us it's hard to imagine how professional caregivers can provide empathy and care to patients day in and day out. They represent the majority of people in the medical profession, and their acts are in total contrast to the negative bedside manner that some patients experience. In fact, many family caregivers said that it was acts of kindness from the staff that actually drew them into personal relationships with them.

The job of professional caregivers is to give high quality and safe care to your patient, improve the odds of survival and recovery, and help restore his quality of life. While they are charged with tremendous responsibility, they're also just people. To the degree that you, as a non-professional but devoted and dedicated caregiver, can establish positive and constructive relationships with them, your patient will be even better served, and you'll find it easier to do your job as an advocate.

## Letting the Patient Call the Shots

Many of the caregivers interviewed talked about the challenge of allowing the patient to make the key decisions, even when they disagreed with the patient's preferences:

**Abby's sister** *As a new caregiver, the hardest thing for me was knowing that I had to live with her answer about which way we were going and whether she would accept treatment —letting her decide whether she lived or died. You do your best, but you're not going through the illness yourself. It's their decision in the end.*

99

**Debbie B's husband** *You're not going to be able to control this cancer or the way your loved one deals with it. It's between him and the disease. You're there to support the person who's battling the disease, but you're not there to change the dynamic. You can't change the outcome. As a patient, Debbie very much wanted to be in control.*

Sometimes letting patients make their own decisions is very challenging, especially when they seem to be doing self-destructive things. This happened to **Patti's daughter** after her mother received a lung cancer diagnosis:

*She wasn't shocked by the diagnosis. She kept smoking and said, "Let me enjoy my last year." I was frustrated by that because it made me feel she wasn't trying as hard as I was to help her stay alive. But I didn't want arguing to be my last experience with her. Yes, I voiced my concern, but it wasn't worth getting angry with her about it.*

It was just as challenging for **Sharon's sister** when Sharon was suffering from metastatic breast cancer and engaged in religious "healing" activities that seemed to deplete her energy and were doing little medical good:

*Sharon felt embraced by the people at the church. I resented them for making her feel that if she just jumped through enough hoops and tried hard enough, God would heal her. I supported her even if I didn't agree. She had nothing else. She felt the need to do something, and maybe it helped her keep fighting. Is that the kind of God we have?*

*If it's working for the patient, the caregiver has to let it happen. It's a gift not to drain their energy trying to talk them out of something that you don't support. Emotional, psychological, and spiritual considerations are as important as physical ones, and they may even take precedence at times.*

As much as you may love the patient, it's not your body, spirit, or soul that's being attacked by the cancer. By letting him "call the shots," you're showing your affection and support. If his decision is doing something that will counteract the benefits of his medical treatment, by all means speak up and ensure that your patient's oncologist has been informed. But if whatever he's doing is something that gives him hope and doesn't impede effective treatment, it's not worth disagreeing.

## Keeping Hope Alive

Hope. It's a curious thing. It's about belief in the possible. It's about refusing to give up. It's about persisting in the face of adversity, even when the odds and the facts seem to be working against you. It's what helps you make the best of a difficult situation.

For some caregivers, like **Tiffany's husband**, the role of attitude manager comes naturally, but that doesn't mean it's easy:

> *The hardest thing was being the positive voice and always saying if you get through chemo, you'll be fine. You have to maintain a positive voice, and not let the patient get caught in the realization of his own mortality. Constantly talk about the future and build positive thinking. Keep the day-to-day stuff away, and be the go-between and the filter.*

For **Judy M's husband**, staying positive meant following Judy's lead during her bout with metastasized breast cancer. Like Tiffany, she provided the steady rock that kept the couple focused:

> *She wanted to live at all costs, so that helped me stay strong and supportive through all of it. She had the gritty determination to beat it and to do whatever it took. I gained strength by following her lead. I learned for the first time that you can't deny the pain and emotional turmoil and anxiety that the other person is going through. I could only acknowledge that I couldn't make it better, so the best thing to do was just be there.*

Some caregivers play mind games to stay positive. For example, **René's wife** described choosing which parts of the available information they would work with and what parts they would ignore in order to maintain their optimism:

> *When we saw the oncologist, he said that René probably had about two or three years to live. That was really devastating. The facts he gave were tough, so we decided to ignore them, because he didn't say that was true in 100% of the cases. Whatever the low percentage is who live longer, we decided that we'd be in it. Now we're at four years, so it's working.*

Now, nine years after his diagnosis, René continues to thrive.

Sometimes caregivers set their minds toward constructive coping when they'd seen others who didn't deal with losses gracefully. After seeing her mother handle her father's death in a negative way, it was no surprise that **Carl's wife**, a retired social work case manager, wasn't about to take his residual challenges after a partial leg amputation as a permanent restriction on their lives:

> *We both feel a real loss of things we loved doing, like mountain climbing and hiking, but we have new things or things we do more of now. I pushed Carl to know that he didn't need two legs to swim. He had been a very good swimmer, and it was so normalizing for him. I told him all he needed was his torso and arms. He couldn't control losing his leg, but he could control what he does with the rest of him. We just applied our own optimism; instinctively we wanted to get on with it and not get stuck.*

Now Carl is swimming again and feeling both confident and competent in doing so.

Hope was critically important to many of the caregivers:

> **Brian's wife** *Brian has been pretty upbeat since he realized there is a chance and hope for a cure. Now we know the track the treatment will be taking, so we're hanging on to a rainbow. Without that, nothing else matters.*

> **Rob's wife** *I had had a meltdown before the biopsy was done regarding the fact that the tumor was wrapped around Rob's carotid artery and he could have a stroke. Then I read about a guy who was killed when his all-terrain vehicle*

*flipped over. I looked at Rob and I realized he's here right now, and he has a chance, and he feels good, so I can't dwell on poor me when people can lose a loved one in a flash.*

**Tom's wife** *You have to plan to live, and whatever happens, happens. There's a poem called "The Dash."[23] When you see a tombstone and it has the date of birth and a dash and the date of death, it's not when you were born or when you died that matters, but it's what you did in the middle. You have to have hope, and you have to keep living life.*

Overall, staying positive is often about keeping your perspective. Cancer is tough stuff. There's no doubt about that. These remarks may sound like Pollyanna speaking, but caregivers offered them in all sincerity, knowing they fought their way through the dark to reach these conclusions. No one knows how many of their loved ones will survive, but all of them are marching forward determined to keep their eyes on the blessings they still have. Most caregivers found that such an attitude helped both patient and caregiver to heal and to make the most of their lives while fighting one battle at a time.

---

23 *www.lindaellis.net.*

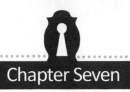

# Chapter Seven

# Resources for the Journey

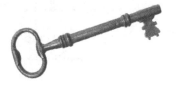

The cancer journey is likely to be full of challenges. Some you can anticipate—how to cope with family and friends wanting to be involved, for example. Others may come unexpectedly along the way—a crisis, a setback, a treatment available only in another state. Usually, there is less time to plan at that point than most of us would prefer, but there are a surprising number and variety of resources you can call on for help, if you know where to look. For example, while nine-year-old Lanie was spending extended periods in a leading children's research hospital, her mother didn't learn until months later that she could have had vouchers to help pay for her parking, food, and gasoline. The hospital didn't volunteer that information, and she didn't know to ask.

Like Lanie's mother, many of the interviewees who contributed to this book discovered the resources they needed *after* the fact, in some cases too late to take advantage of them. As a result, this was one of the major clusters of "things I wish I'd known" that caregivers identified.

This chapter provides an overview of seven types of resources. Additional resources are provided on the website *www.thingsiwishidknown.com*, on the Resources tab:

**Patient Navigators for the Health Care System**

**Social Workers and Other Mental Health Professionals**

**Reality Checks from Other Patients and Caregivers**

**Sharing Information with Family and Friends**

**Coordinating Help from Others**

**Finding Free Lodging for Treatment Away from Home**

**Finding Resources for the Long-Distance Caregiver**

## Patient Navigators for the Health Care System

For novices, the encounter with the various aspects of the health care system—from medical terminology to hospital procedures to post-surgery or treatment options—can be overwhelming. You don't know the ground rules, whom to approach, or what questions to ask, and you have no idea what help you'll need or want. **Jen P's husband** described this problem:

> *The whole process of going through the health care system was new to us. What's involved and how do you do it? There's no guidebook about how to work through the medical system—the administrative stuff, whom to call, who does what.*

It isn't always easy to find out from your doctor and hospital what resources for support beyond medical care are available. Fortunately, there may be one very useful, all-around personal resource you can call on early in the process: an education and support specialist called a patient navigator.

This relatively new position in the health care field was created to help individual cancer patients access appropriate services and support from the health care system, government bodies, and the community. According to the American Cancer Society, in 2009 there were more than 700 patient navigators in hospitals across the country, around 130 of them sponsored by the Society and its funding partners. The Commission on Cancer will be phasing in standards for patient navigators as a criterion for cancer program certification beginning in 2015.

Each navigator works on a confidential basis to help patients access:

- ❧ Information about treatment options, management of side effects, and so on

- ❧ Information about what is available to caregivers from the hospital, including parking support, gas subsidies, meal vouchers, support groups, and classes

- ❧ Language interpreter services

- ❧ Billing, insurance, and financial assistance

- ❧ Physical therapy

- ❧ Nutrition counseling

- ❧ Home health assistance

- ❧ Survivorship information

Patient navigators also help patients understand and adhere to their prescribed medication schedules, track follow-up visit appointments, and find rides to treatment. If you would like to avail yourself of such help, ask your hospital whether it has a patient navigator, and be sure to contact him or her *early on* so you don't miss out on any benefits.

There is no question that patient navigators improve the outcomes for their patients. The first patient navigator program was launched at Harlem Hospital in New York City in 1990. Between 1995 and 2000, five-year cancer survival rates improved there from 39% to 70%, and diagnoses of late-stage cancers in Harlem dropped from 40% to 21%. The pilot program was so successful that it became the basis for the 2005 Patient Navigator and Chronic Disease Act.

For more information or to find a navigator to help you, there are two efficient resources:

- ❧ The website of the American Society of Clinical Oncologists (*www.cancer.net/patient*)

- ❧ The American Cancer Society at 800-ACS-2345 or go to *www.cancer.org*

## Social Workers and Other Mental Health Professionals

Knowing when stress is becoming too hard to handle and when you and/or your patient would benefit from some form of counseling is an important coping behavior for all caregivers. It's not a sign of weakness to ask to see a social worker, visit a psychiatrist, or participate in a support group. On the contrary, it's an indication of strength that you can recognize your vulnerability and understand how important it is to reach out to others during a time of crisis.

While a patient navigator provides informational support, the social worker offers guidance and counsel in managing communication and relationships with the hospital's medical staff and in handling personal relationships affected by the cancer experience. It may be a good idea to ask about what mental health professional resources are available when you first visit the hospital during a diagnostic or pre-surgical process. Many of the leading cancer centers, especially teaching and/or research institutions, have such resources on site and available within the clinical department where your patient is being treated.

Many hospitals maintain a cadre of professionals licensed by their respective state who hold a Masters in Social Work (MSW) degree and have received additional clinical training about how cancer treatments affect both patient and caregivers. This dual focus allows hospital-based social workers to develop insights about day-to-day challenges as well as long-term issues.

**Mike S's wife** found the social worker invaluable when she and her husband were told that his pancreatic cancer was terminal and they thought he had only weeks to live:

> *Our first visit was with a medical oncologist and a surgeon. Our adult children came with us. The surgeon said he couldn't operate. On the same day, I had also made an appointment to see an oncology social worker. It was a good move. We entered her tiny office and met a professional who was kind, experienced, and understanding. Our family felt safe acknowledging that our world had changed forever. We*

*had a trained listener for safe conversation. We all cried. It helped to share our feelings about how each of us was in such pain. It was good for Mike to see the impact it was having for his young adult children. It started us on a positive track for handling the disease together as a family.*

This talented and caring social worker helped guide them through a process that extended Mike's life by more than two years and brought the family peace during the process.

Social workers may also serve as intermediaries among doctors, patients, and caregivers, and participate in some of the medical appointments. For example, **Tim N's wife** pointed out:

*The social worker was really helpful. When we didn't understand, he'd find out the information or go with us to facilitate conversation with the oncologist to get answers to our questions.*

**Debbie B's husband** found the support of the social worker invaluable as he and Debbie navigated the extremes of the medical system to try to save her life:

*The notion that it would be very helpful to have a social worker involved with your medical care is so important. He made all the difference in the world in her care. He'd come to appointments with us when there were difficult issues to deal with. He was on the core team. In terms of medical care, the first thing that comes to mind is his role, especially toward the end.*

Social workers focus on helping individuals, couples, and families to deal with emotional and relationship issues in both personalized settings and support groups. They tend to be most helpful in the more serious or complicated cancer cases. Social workers often organize information that will help you to make treatment decisions, participate in meetings with the medical team where treatment options are discussed, and help you cope with the shift you may experience in your traditional roles, responsibilities, and relationships as you take on major caregiving activities.

Key topics that social workers address may include:[24]

- ⟡ Handling employment issues, such as rights under the Family Medical Leave Act and how to communicate with the patient's or your own employer to maintain your job under changed conditions.

- ⟡ Preparing children for anticipated changes in family life.

- ⟡ Providing relationship counseling, including issues of sexuality and intimacy, the impact of cancer on reproductive abilities, and family disagreements about the course of treatment.

- ⟡ Coping with survivor issues, including whether the cancer will return.

- ⟡ Managing differences between the patient and caregiver in attitudes toward various courses of treatment (which often reflect differences within a family, especially when children live at a distance or have been affected by the divorce or death of their other parent).

- ⟡ Deciding how and when to seek palliative care (relief of pain).

- ⟡ Managing expectations toward the end of life.

- ⟡ Determining how and when to seek hospice services.

Some social workers interact with the patient and caregiver over a period of years and become trusted resources and friends long after the cancer episode has passed.

## Reality Checks from Other Patients and Caregivers

Some patients and caregivers find it useful to join support groups where they can learn from others who are going through the same experience or just want to share their feelings. These kinds of support groups are generally available through hospitals and their cancer centers free of charge.

---

24 For definitions, see *www.cancer.org/Treatment.*

Overcoming the inevitable loneliness that is part of the cancer journey can ease anxiety and offer a reality check. For example, shortly after her four-year-old son was diagnosed with a brain tumor, **Michael L's mother** met another mother whose child was in the midst of successful treatment for a brain tumor:

> *The night the pathology report was coming back, another little boy and his mother were in the room. She asked whether things were OK. My father said, "I'm really sorry, but we just found out that my grandson has a brain tumor, so we can't talk." She said, "Oh, my son has a brain tumor too."*
>
> *After I came back with the pathology report, my father introduced me to her. I fell into her lap, and she allowed me to cry for an hour. She's become my best friend. Fate brought us together that night. Knowing they were farther along in the process really helped. Somebody else had gone through the same nightmare.*

It didn't make the nightmare go away, but it gave Michael's mom a strong shoulder to lean on when things got rough during treatment. Both children are thriving today, and their mothers continue to be friends.

Other patients and caregivers have found virtual communities where they can exchange concerns and suggestions with others. One of these is the ACS's Cancer Survivors Network (CSN) (*www.csn.cancer.org*). The Society defines a cancer patient as a survivor from the moment of diagnosis, so CSN serves both those who are still in the midst of treatment and those whose treatment is finished. The site offers email services, discussion boards, and chat rooms on topics of concern to its members and gives people the opportunity to connect with those who have undergone similar experiences.

A second such resource for networking is the Cancer Hope Network (*www.cancerhopenetwork.org*) which can be reached at 800-552-4366.

There are websites that offer similar networking and discussion opportunities within a particular cancer "family." For example, **Richard's wife** found a lymphoma discussion group on Facebook:

*I was searching for people with mantle cell lymphoma, and I ended up talking to and befriending a guy who went through it. Knowing about his experience has helped. It's a rare form of cancer, so for me, it helped to talk about it with someone else who was going through it.*

**Tom's wife** is using several sources as networking tools that also tell her where to find other specialized support groups:

*The website, www.ACOR.org, represents every cancer. You can go to lists of diagnoses, and you can access different treatment options. The Liddy Shriver Foundation and the Sarcoma Alliance are also good places to go for information. They allow posting and replies, or emailing back and forth, or exchanging posts. I found these resources to be useful, both at the information stage and now. For rare cancers, there aren't usually good support resources locally.*

Finally, the American Cancer Society offers various useful links at *www.cancer.org/Treatment* to a variety of local resources, including support groups for breast and prostate cancers, rides to treatment, and help coping with hair loss and other side effects from cancer treatments. It also provides access to links for finding free lodging, a topic covered beginning on page 117.

The people and resources that can help you avoid having to learn the ropes through trial and error can save you time, energy, and frustration. You're not weak if you accept such guidance, support, or help. In fact, you're making a smart choice that will ease your journey so you'll have more energy for the fight ahead and can focus on easing your loved one's quality of life during treatment. You're also providing a welcome outlet for people who've experienced the stress of a cancer diagnosis and just want to make your life a little easier during a tough period.

## Sharing Information with Family and Friends

Some patients and caregivers find sharing information about cancer difficult at first, considering illness a private matter. For others it comes naturally. **Judy M's husband**, a recovering alcoholic, knew the importance of having a support network with whom he and Judy could talk about challenging issues:

> *We were very open about it. I never hid my alcoholism at all, so it was easy to share information about her cancer. It's not productive or useful or advantageous to keep it a family secret. Judy and I talked openly about it, and we projected confidence, strength, and faith. Our strength helped our friends be stronger in their support. We set the tone for them.*

Sometimes patients and caregivers who were raised to be independent and self-sufficient find the idea of asking for help difficult to accept. They can't imagine being in a situation they can't handle on their own. **Annie's husband** was not unique when he said, *I'm more of a giver than a taker*, to explain why he didn't accept help easily.

Similarly, **Rob's wife** commented:

> *People would ask me, "How are you doing?" but I felt it would be selfish to be honest and say how I was really doing. It was hard to accept the help, like money from fund raisers. I know they were being generous, but sometimes it felt like we had become some of those people who always needed help.*

Like Annie's husband and Rob's wife, some of us just try to "power through it" when faced with an obstacle, hoping that we'll be able to regain control if we just keep motoring forward. It always worked in the past, so why wouldn't it work now just as well? The message from the interviewed caregivers is very simple: *Get real, and get over it.* Letting other people help is nothing to be ashamed of. Cancer isn't just a bump or a scratch, or a detour in a normal day. It is unexpected, life-changing, and scary. It alters your world view, your sense of self, and your perspective on what matters. No patient or caregiver should have to go through that experience alone.

Your friends, neighbors, and work associates want to help. They're glad they're not going through what you are. Letting them help is a gift to them, but it's important to figure out how to avoid being overwhelmed by offers.

## Coordinating Help from Others

You may be surprised at the number of people who want to help or will call to ask what they can do to help you. Such generous offers may be a mixed blessing, however. Several caregivers—**Judy O's husband**, for example—said that the sheer number of people they had to get back to by phone or email caused them considerable stress:

> *I kept telling myself I should be able to do this, but the phone calls were annoying because I had to return them. I'd get 10 messages at night asking ,"How's Judy?," and I'd have to call every person back and repeat the same thing at night when I was emotionally exhausted.*

**Tiffany's husband** felt the same way:

> *It is an overwhelming and tiring experience. You want people to call and express support, but the hard part about the phone calls is that when I got home, I had to return them.*

Lynn recognized that her cancer would cause her husband an enormous communications challenge, so she set up her own system. According to **Lynn's husband**:

> *Before she went to the hospital, she set up an email list and taught me how to do email. I'd send a nightly blast to 20 or so friends and family. I can write, so I could give a realistic picture without seeming too bleak.*

When **Mike S's wife** set up her own communications system, she discovered an extra benefit—it helped her organize her thoughts and feelings:

> *In the beginning, people in the community knew things about Mike's situation much too soon. It seemed like gossip to me. So I set up what I called the "jungle drum." I'd send out an email to our friends and family. It was therapeutic for me to*

*put the information down in writing and make it clear and accurate. People could also leave messages for Mike without expecting a return call. That let Mike listen to the good wishes, especially when he was in the hospital.*

There are several coordination tools available today on the Internet, each with different strengths and limitations. **Carole's husband** created LotsaHelpingHands (*www.lotsahelpinghands.com*), a coordination tool that allows the patient and his caregivers to specify what they could use and when. Anyone who has the log-in information can register to see the patient updates, sign up for providing rides or delivering meals, and offer other kinds of support to the patient and his family.

**Kathy**, a serial caregiver, is on her third round of supporting a cancer patient (her father Jim, her father-in-law Artie, and now her sister Deb). She relies on this website for both communication and coordination:

*LotsaHelpingHands is wonderful. It has a calendar that's color-coded for when you can sign up to bring meals and who has already signed up for what meal. I wrote the narrative and told people what was going on. Then we sent the link to everyone in our address book, and to her boss and her co-workers, and they sent it out. We can also do fund raising on the site under the resources tab. My husband opened a bank account for the money raised.*

*Within three days, 41 people had already joined the website. It has their contacts and their information. I can tell who has signed in and who hasn't. I have to give people permission to join. People can send well wishes and can use the color-coded schedule to sign up for bringing meals, giving the kids rides to their commitments, or giving gift cards or financial donations.*

**Jenn S** and her husband are fans of *www.CaringBridge.com*:

*One of the hardest things besides actually making the decisions is having the same conversation over and over and over with people. The same message about what it is and what*

> *we're going to do, 40 times. To deal with that, we did use CaringBridge and still do. She's up to something like 51,000 hits on it. It's one of the most useful things I've encountered.*
>
> *You can do it now right from your iPhone sitting in the hospital. It makes it easier to get the word out. It was good for her once she came out the other side to be able to sit back and see that support and read people saying how much they cared about her.*

**Steve's wife** found *www.carepages.com* to be helpful, especially for exchanging messages with friends and relatives about patient updates.

Mindy, who was diagnosed with stage IV metastatic melanoma in her lungs and liver with no primary site ever found, was in a clinical trial that took her halfway across the country for three months. To help handle the impact of her chemo and her absences from home, a friend registered the family on *www.takethemameal.com*, which focuses almost exclusively on food arrangements. **Mindy's husband** says:

> *Their website is a useful tool for specifying dinner hours, family likes and dislikes, days you'd like to receive a meal, and directions to the house. People we know or were connected to would list what they were bringing and their phone number. A friend set it up for us five months in advance. There are also hints about bringing paper plates, bringing some breakfast items, and so on. It was really helpful because there were fewer phone calls, explanations, and even emails about the subject.*

One of the newest websites that focuses on helping cancer patients and caregivers organize their supporters is My Cancer Circle. It was created by Boehringer Ingelheim Pharmaceuticals, Inc. in collaboration with CancerCare, and powered by Lotsa Helping Hands. The website helps coordinate volunteer activities and provides a space for private dialogue among community members, patient updates, and offers to give caregivers a break (*mycancercircle.lotsahelpinghands.com/caregiving/home/*).

Online tools like these make it far easier to let others provide you with tangible help.

## Finding Free Lodging for Treatment Away from Home

In this age of increasing specialization, cancer patients may need to travel considerable distances to receive the kind of treatment most suited to their particular cancer. As a result, one of the most costly "collateral" expenses can be lodging while your patient is receiving outpatient treatment in a city far from home. Fortunately, there are a number of resources for free lodging throughout the country, and more are popping up each year. Four of these are described below.

### Hope Lodge (American Cancer Society)

(*www.cancer.org/Treatment* and search "Hope Lodge")

As of early 2012, there were 31 Hope Lodges operating across the country and several others under construction. According to the website, "In general, Hope Lodge is available to patients and caregivers actively undergoing cancer treatment on an outpatient basis. Patients must live at least 40 miles or a one-hour drive time away from the treatment facility. Priority is given to patients needing three or more nights of lodging. Patients must be at least 18 years old (exceptions are made at some locations) and be independently mobile in the event of an emergency. Patients are not screened for any financial or demographic criteria."

Each Hope Lodge is different, but all offer private suites and private bathroom facilities that can accommodate an adult patient and a caregiver. Common areas include full kitchens, laundry facilities, cancer resource rooms, and places for quiet reflection. Some lodges have entertainment rooms, computer rooms, libraries, and other special purpose rooms which can be used for shared craft activities or to host visiting musicians or other entertainers. The kitchen facilities offer separate food storage locations but provide opportunities for interaction if and when the patient and caregiver choose.

117

Interviewees who had stayed at Hope Lodges were effusive in their compliments. They said they had made lifelong friends and received important support from people who understood what they were going through. More importantly, they said that they didn't have to talk about their cancers if they didn't want to, and that the environment felt *just like home.*

There is generally a waiting list for admission, but often the hospital will make contact with the appropriate Hope Lodge on behalf of the patient to schedule rooms to coincide with treatment dates. If you think you'll need this kind of lodging, let your medical team know early on. To find the Hope Lodge closest to your hospital, go online or call 800-ACS-2345. If there is not a Hope Lodge in your area, your local ACS office may have negotiated other free or discounted places to stay. Call 800-ACS-2345 for more information.

### Joe's House (*www.joeshouse.org/Lodging*)

This website has drop-down menus for each state and for the hospital where your patient will be treated. A list will pop up showing both discounted hotel arrangements and free lodging sites, together with contact information and pricing. The negotiated discounted hotel arrangements may vary by hospital.

### National Association of Hospital Hospitality Homes
(*www.nahhh.org*)

This is a nationwide association of over 200 nonprofit organizations that provide lodging and support services to patients and caregivers receiving medical treatment far from their homes. Most of the lodging is less costly than hotels, and some is free. In addition to helping patients and caregivers find lodging, NAHHH works to expand medical lodging options in under-served communities and shares best practices throughout its network. Members include Hope Lodges, Ronald McDonald Houses, and the Veterans' Administration's Fisher House Program. Check out the website or call 800-542-9730.

## Finding Resources for the Long-Distance Caregiver

A few of the interviewees had looked after patients who lived a distance away from them. Caregivers who lived far away tended to come for periodic visits and were less involved in the day-to-day medical aspects of caregiving. In such situations, there is often a need for a surrogate or other professional services to fill in for medical and household caregiving activities.

Frieda was 90 years old when she was diagnosed with multiple myeloma. She had been a ballroom dancer until recently, so she was in fairly good physical condition. A first-generation American, she grew up during the Depression, expressed little emotion, and shared hardly any information about her health with family members. **Frieda's daughter**, who lived a three-hour drive away, discovered that there were many local resources to help out-of-town caregivers:

> *I called the social worker at the local senior center, and she gave me several names and numbers. I found an RN, Mary, who was in business with an attorney helping long-distance caregivers. She stood in for me when I couldn't be there and helped me find a home health aide agency to give 24-hour nursing care. Mom understood that she needed it. Again, Mary helped me to do interviews, and she found a young woman who was inexperienced but sweet and who cared. It worked out well.*

**George's daughter Kathy** was more directly involved when her 72-year-old father, who lived a plane-ride away, was diagnosed with pancreatic cancer. The situation was complicated by the fact that George, a Chinese immigrant, didn't always understand or follow through on his doctor's instructions. The solution for Kathy and her sister, who lived closer, was to rely on local family friends and to generate an email trail. That allowed them to convey information back and forth so they could take turns following up on their father's situation and at the same time create a record for later reference:

119

*We had a really good family friend who was a nurse and could explain things to my father. I'd fly out to meet with his surgeon every couple of weeks because I knew Dad didn't know what was going on and what to expect. Because we talked to him so regularly and he felt so supported, he would listen to us. I also have a very good friend who is a surgeon at UCLA, and Dad knew we were constantly talking with her to help us understand what to expect. We filtered some things, but we had a resource that was quite valuable.*

The number of long-distance caregivers among interviewees was relatively small, but what they had learned and their resulting messages were clear:

- Make an initial visit to meet the doctor and to talk about both your patient's health situation and how involved you plan to be in his care. Be there for critical events like surgery and first and last radiation or chemo treatments, especially if the patient is elderly, unlikely to advocate for himself, or will benefit from the presence of a younger, more assertive caregiver.

- Ensure that you have a direct communications channel with your patient's physicians and that your loved one approves of your receiving periodic updates from them. That way, if questions or unusual situations arise, you'll be in the loop and can help make decisions. It may require your patient signing HIPAA paperwork to authorize you to have access to relevant information. In the meantime, seek out local caregiving surrogates who can fill in for you at medical appointments, support household needs, and keep you informed about the progress your patient is making during treatments.

- Think of ways you can simplify the logistics of your patient's living situation—anything from finding someone to mow the lawn to arranging for periodic delivery of flowers or a prepared meal.

❧ If the patient is a parent and you have siblings, have an explicit conversation with them about how you and they will divide caregiving and other responsibilities. Determine the degree to which your patient will be able to manage financial matters during his illness, especially with the influx of additional paperwork (bills and insurance statements) for medical and other new services. If help is going to be needed with record-keeping or in the processing of bills for payment, set up a system early to address evolving insurance, legal, and financial issues and for providing that help so that bills will be paid on time and records will be complete. If a durable power of attorney is likely to be needed, get it executed right away.

❧ Don't feel guilty about any choices you make regarding how frequently you can be there in person. We all do our best, and many of us don't have the choice of opting out of work or home responsibilities to offer full-time caregiving in a distant location.

Some of the advice about long-distance caregiving contrasts with earlier lessons that suggest letting the patient make his own decisions. When dealing with the elderly, you have to make a judgment about how well they can manage their own care, especially if they don't seem to understand, aren't being candid about their condition, or seem to be moving in directions that counter good medical advice. In such cases, you have to step in to ensure the best quality of life for them, even if you have to do it at a distance.

# Chapter Eight

# Managing Financial and Legal Issues

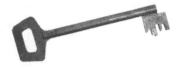

If you thought medical bills were high before your encounter with cancer, fasten your seatbelt. There are a number of financial issues you may have to face, depending on the type of cancer and treatment. For example, your patient may need to travel away from home to access the right treatment, so you may be faced with travel, food, and lodging costs. Similarly, bone marrow transplants will require extended absences from work, so verifying the terms of a medical leave with your respective employers and the implications for insurance coverage become essential. As a caregiver, you are the most likely person to have the time, energy and perspective to make sure the monetary aspects of the journey are well under control.

To manage the overall financial impact of cancer, a particularly useful resource is a booklet entitled "Frankly Speaking About Cancer," which is available through The Cancer Support Community in either download or print format.[25]

---

25 *www.cancersupportcommunity.org.* If you prefer to order a hard copy of this publication, write to The Cancer Support Community, 1050 17th Street, NW, Suite 500, Washington, DC 20036 (phone: 202-659-9709, 1-888-793-9355).

It deals with:

- ≪ How to gather needed information from the whole range of possible providers who might be involved in your patient's care

- ≪ Health insurance issues (including private insurance, COBRA,[26] Medicare, Medicaid, and communicating with your insurance company)

- ≪ Employment and disability, income, and debt

- ≪ Prescription medication costs

- ≪ Medicare and Medicaid, Social Security, and co-pay assistance.

Some of these topics and other, more specialized resources are covered in greater detail in the following four sections:

**Household Record-keeping**

**Insurance Issues**

**Employment and Other Legal Issues**

**The Cost of Prescription Drugs**

Note: This chapter includes a great deal of information and many resource references. You may want to skim through these sections so you become familiar with what's here and can differentiate items you want to learn about now from those you'll want to revisit later, when the particular issue is more timely.

## Household Record-keeping

Regardless of the complexity or severity of the cancer diagnosis, record-keeping is critical to streamlining the processes of filing insurance claims, keeping income tax records for medical expenses (including mileage), and making sure that ongoing bills get paid along the way.

---

26  COBRA insurance (named for the Consolidated Omnibus Budget Reconciliation Act) is insurance that you can purchase for a limited period through an employer after employment ends.

**Kathy** is one of our serial caregivers. After her three experiences taking care of her father, father-in-law, and sister, she had a number of recommendations for others who find themselves in her shoes:

> *Check everything. Don't assume that your insurance covers everything. Check on when it expires, and check your state health care regulations. Check every policy. My sister will lose her health insurance because her job will only pay it for six months. She can buy COBRA, but it will cost $1,500 per month. There's a state insurance program in each state. She may qualify for SSDI,[27] too, while she's going through it. Always check into the notices when you get them from insurers or from Medicare. Watch out that they aren't giving you expiration notices.*

This means opening the envelope from any insurance carrier or medical provider when it comes, rather than letting the mail stack up until there's more time to go through it. Chances are, you won't get more time, and the one envelope you fail to open and review may be something that's critical to your patient's continued insurance coverage. One caregiver didn't open what looked like a routine mailing and ended up missing a Medicare enrollment deadline, which resulted in having to pay full costs for her patient's medical expenses until the following year's enrollment period.

**Kathy** also suggested:

> *Between the co-pays and the changes in prescriptions, you have to keep things organized. Create a medical bills filing system that you can use to keep track of what's been paid and what hasn't. Prepare to match the explanations of benefits from the insurer to the bills, and keep a log that allows you to track what's come in when, what's been paid and when, what's the balance owed by the patient, and so on.*

Bills are not going to be bundled in a way that makes sense to a patient or caregiver; they're bundled for the convenience of the health care provider.

---

27  SSDI refers to Social Security Disability Insurance, which may be available after filing with the Social Security Administration in your local area.

Each individual who contributed to a particular treatment may bill separately. For example, a surgical procedure may incur separate bills from the hospital (for the operating room and supplies), the surgeon, and the anesthesiologist. You may think that because a certain procedure took place on a particular date at a specific location, all bills should arrive together. In reality, they will come at different times and from providers whose names you won't recognize because they are mailed from billing companies unfamiliar to you. You'll need to verify and track these by date and place of service to make sense of them.

**Kathy** further suggested:

> *Record your mileage and parking costs on all medical visits for tax deductions. Each may be small, but they can really add up over time.*
>
> *Keep a list of all of the household bills that are paid online, together with the website, log-in name and passwords, credit card number used for each, and so on. This will allow you or another member of the caregiving team to ensure that regular bills are being paid on time.*

Finally, **Kathy** recommended that caregivers set up a separate bank account for grouping outlays associated with cancer treatment, especially if the charges are for a person who is not normally a member of your household.

## Insurance Issues

Insurance issues can be as complex as medical ones, if not more so. From coverage of procedures and prescription drugs to how a cancer diagnosis will affect the patient's work life, there are a host of potential pitfalls to avoid.

The 2010 Affordable Care Act (ACA) was intended to phase in over time and has significant implications for lifetime insurance limits, coverage of pre-existing conditions, insurance coverage for children until age 26 under parents' insurance plans, and a variety of other access and coverage issues for cancer patients. The act faced political and judicial challenges at many levels from the day it was passed. Regardless of how the law is changed or implemented, your first step should be to check your patient's insurance policy to determine what kinds of services are covered and whether any important ones are not. Then, for the ones that are, determine what qualifiers exist regarding the settings in which they are covered, and at what reimbursement level. Check coverage down to the level of the individual practitioner: for example, different radiation oncologists in the same imaging center may have applied a different code to their various places of business, thereby qualifying one location for coverage from a particular insurance carrier and disqualifying another.

Considering the various political and judicial pressures being exerted to either challenge or de-fund the ACA, you should take nothing for granted.

In addition, remember if the patient is under the age of 65 and has received Social Security or Railroad Retirement Board disability benefits for 24 months or is in end-stage Renal Disease, he may be eligible for coverage through Medicare. You can check eligibility rules at *www.medicare. gov.* Low-income patients may be eligible for Medicaid (*www.medicaid. gov*), depending on your state's eligibility guidelines.

### Reviewing the Patient's Insurance Policy

In light of the issues caregivers described regarding insurance coverage, there are routine questions you'll want to get answered when you review your patient's policy:[28]

- ❧ How long will the patient be covered? Will there be a need to renew during the treatment period?

- ❧ What will insurance pay for?

- ❧ Does the doctor's office (or do I) need to call the insurance company before each treatment in order to qualify for insurance reimbursement? How often and under what circumstances will the patient or his doctors need to get pre-authorizations?

---

28  For a more comprehensive list of questions, see
    *www.cancer.net/all-about-cancer/managing-cost-cancer-care.*

~& What will the patient have to pay for directly, beyond what insurance covers?

~& Can we see any doctor we want, or do we need to choose from a list of preferred providers?

~& Does the patient need a written referral to see a specialist once he's been diagnosed with cancer?

~& Is there a co-pay (required out-of-pocket payment) for each appointment? If so, how much?

~& Is there a deductible (certain amount the patient needs to pay) before insurance pays anything?

~& Where should we get prescription drugs? Do we need to use mail order or can we go to a pharmacy? Which costs less? Will drugs obtained through the hospital be reimbursed?

~& Does insurance pay for all tests and treatments, regardless of whether delivered on an inpatient or an outpatient basis?

All of these questions can be answered either by reading the policy itself or by calling the insurance carrier's customer service line.

## Dealing With Insurance and Medical Debt Problems

There are several good information resources to guide you in handling health insurance issues. Start with a hospital cancer patient navigator. Then check out three organizations that can help.

One is the American Cancer Society website *(www.cancer.org)*, which offers good background information. After searching "paying for treatment" on the website, you will find several tabs dealing with insurance and financial issues as well as how to handle insurance claim denials and locate treatment resources.

The second is the Patient Advocate Foundation (PAF) *(www.patient-advocate.org)*, which provides negotiation, mediation, and arbitration services free of charge to resolve access-to-healthcare issues for insured, uninsured, and under-insured patients diagnosed with chronic, debilitating, and life-threatening conditions. PAF professionals also seek to preserve employment and resolve medical debt crisis issues that threaten to delay prescribed health care services. The organization gives information about clinical trials, offers help with finding co-pay assistance in each state, and provides counseling about how to negotiate payment plans with medical providers. A report on its website lists contact information for other organizations—both national and by state—that provide financial assistance. PAF has partnerships with the American Cancer Society, Lance Armstrong Foundation LiveStrong, Susan G. Komen for the Cure, The Leukemia & Lymphoma Society, Centers for Disease Control, and others.

Third, if you have any questions or problems regarding insurance coverage or medical debt, contact the Ombudsman at the Center for Medicare and Medicaid Services by phoning 800-MEDICARE and asking to be transferred to the Ombudsman or by going to the website *www.cms.gov*.

## Dealing with Disruptions in Insurance Coverage

Insurance companies don't always have a patient's best interests at heart. Sometimes they refuse to cover certain procedures. Sometimes people lose their health insurance even though they remain eligible. Sometimes the problem is simply a paperwork glitch. The term for that situation is "insurance churning." The Affordable Care Act was intended in part to help cancer patients and their caregivers deal with such issues, but it pays to be vigilant.

Over a year before the ACA was passed, **Trudy's domestic partner** watched in frustration as Trudy jeopardized her life because she had no health insurance:

> *Trudy lost insurance coverage several times. She would have reacted much sooner if she had had insurance, but when she knew she didn't have it, she couldn't put herself or anyone she loved in debt. She was never cured, but her life would be very different now if she had had insurance. Her lack of insurance jeopardized her health.*
>
> *She had 10 lymph nodes removed at the time of the mastectomy, and nine were cancerous. She developed metastatic*

*lumps in nodes on her neck during a period when she wasn't covered by insurance, and she wouldn't go to the doctor because of the expense. So when they got to be the size of an orange, and she hadn't been able to work, a friend in the local community helped her gain access to Social Security Disability Insurance (SSDI). Then right after our state passed an insurance assistance program, she applied and went right away to see the oncologist.*

Churning and the associated risk of interrupted coverage may not disappear even if the ACA remains in effect. That's why you should read the small print in your patient's insurance policies carefully regardless of whether his coverage is in a public or private program. In addition, pay attention to any documentation that you receive that asks whether you want to renew existing coverage or to sign up for a different plan.

Also check with your existing provider to ensure you haven't missed something in the fine print that may mean a recertification date is imminent. The last thing you want is to have the patient lose insurance coverage at a time that might interrupt life-saving treatment.

**René's wife** got immersed in insurance issues while she and her husband were fighting to get him the right treatment for the renal failure that resulted from his multiple myeloma. Her story is instructive for anyone having insurance coverage problems:

*If a procedure or medical visit is rejected by the patient's insurer, talk with the medical team about what additional information or appeal procedure to use next. Sometimes the issue may be as simple as the numerical code that was put on the submission; other times it may be sufficiently complicated that you'll want to consult with the patient navigator or hospital social worker for support and assistance.*

*Also keep in mind that even though you bought insurance with the intent that it would pay for major health expenses if and when they occurred, your insurance company has every financial incentive to reduce the number of claims it pays, so its staff is likely to read the fine print to find grounds on which to reject a claim.*

*At one point René got to be on Medicare, which paid for the dialysis and became his primary insurance. He was participating in a clinical trial to see whether getting a kidney as well as bone marrow from the same donor might make it possible to avoid taking anti-rejection drugs for the rest of his life. At most, his employer's insurance company would only pay 20%. Medicare pays $50,000 a month, or $600,000 a year for dialysis.*

*Part of the time we were fighting both Medicare and the insurance company. As long as his insurance carrier didn't approve its payment share, Medicare wouldn't pay for the kidney transplant. Most people don't have both Medicare and private coverage together, so his case was unique.*

*In October 2009, René's coverage ended, and the insurance company said we had 30 days to appeal the final rejection. I read the information on which the insurance company had based their decision. That's how we found out that his employer had originated a letter to the insurance company saying they should reject our claim. We'd been fighting the insurance company all that time, and it turned out that it was actually his employer that said no. We also discovered that there was a conflicting letter from an independent evaluator for the insurance company who recommended approving the surgery.*

*We got the requested records quickly. We didn't take 'no' for an answer. It's really good that we didn't stop. The timeframe got extended when we filed our appeal, and lo and behold, it got approved months later.*

It took René's wife over four months and countless phone calls to overcome the company's rejection. When I met her, René was recovering from the successful double transplant and doing well.

## Employment and Other Legal Issues

Cancer treatment takes time, and many of us don't have the control to adjust our work schedules around medical commitments. That may lead to employment jeopardy for both cancer patients and their caregivers.

Surprisingly, employment matters weren't a major topic in most of the interviews with caregivers. Some even had bosses enlightened enough to realize that support for their caregiving role represented an investment in a good employee. These employers provided flexibility to juggle work schedules as required to accommodate the patient's medical schedules.

**Michael S's father**, for example, found that his employer was every understanding about the demands that the cancer treatments for his son placed on his time and energies:

> My boss is very supportive of my need to be a caregiver parent and spouse. As a caregiver, they let me work a flexible schedule, and others are willing to cover for me at times. It's part of the company culture. The people I work with took things off my plate so I could deal with family things. Individuals reached out to me.

Unfortunately, not everyone has such a positive experience. The Family Medical Leave Act (FMLA) allows the patient or a family member who is a caregiver to take up to 12 weeks of unpaid leave in the event of serious illness, but only in companies with 50 or more employees. Those interviewees who talked about their workplace difficulties generally were with companies so small that state and federal legislative employee protections didn't apply to them.

**Lanie's mother** used her sick leave and vacation time when her daughter was diagnosed with a serious brain tumor. When Lanie relapsed, she had to take more time off:

> I had been out of work for six weeks, used all my vacation. So I went into work the first day, and at 2 p.m. my mother called and said that Lanie was unconscious. The Family Medical Leave Act had been passed, but my company had less than 50 people and fired me. I couldn't do anything about it.

**Barbara** was her own caregiver. Her treatment for metastasized breast cancer required that she be absent from work from time to time:

> *My employer fired me because I had cancer, but he worded it differently. He said that I missed too many days: "I'm a sole practitioner, and you're my only employee. I can't have you not here." My oncologist said I couldn't go to work. My employer wanted to block me from getting unemployment. He didn't want that cost to be charged back to him.*
>
> *Because he was a sole practitioner, the state and federal disabilities acts didn't apply. The labor attorneys I hired said, "The laws will protect him, and it's a waste of time to try to sue." So we did a negotiated settlement for minor severance pay with an agreement that he couldn't cancel my insurance while I was in treatment.*

There are a number of resources that can help with employment and other legal issues:

- ❧ Patient Advocate Foundation (described on page 124)

- ❧ The Cancer Legal Resource Center (CLRC) is a joint program of the Disability Rights Legal Center and Loyola Law School of Los Angeles. Although based in California, CLRC provides free information and resources *nationwide* on legal issues for patients, survivors, caregivers and employers. These issues include:
  - Employment
  - Medical leave
  - Reasonable workplace accommodations
  - Health insurance
  - Government benefits
  - Patient rights (including genetic discrimination)
  - Insurance: disability insurance, life insurance, Medicare, Medicaid, and Medi-Cal
  - Estate-planning, custody and guardianship, and conservatorship

- Advanced health care directives
- Consumer rights

CLRC is supported by a number of national cancer and legal services organizations. You can reach it by calling either 866-THE-CLRC or 866-843-2572 weekdays between 9 a.m. and 5 p.m. Pacific Standard Time. The intake form is also available online (*www.disabilityrightslegalcenter.org*), and materials are available in both English and Spanish.

∽ A hospital patient navigator, a social worker, or the American Cancer Society's 24-hour multi-lingual help line (800-ACS-2345) may be helpful if the two specialized resources above aren't able to help resolve your issues.

∽ If you are unsure whether an extended leave from work will jeopardize your patient's insurance coverage, you can also check with the U.S. Department of Labor's website at *www.dol.gov* regarding the Family Medical Leave Act (FMLA). In addition, for patients whose cancer is sufficiently advanced that they will not be able to sustain work during treatment, Social Security Disability Insurance (SSDI) may be an important financial resource.

## The Cost of Prescription Drugs

Cancer treatments are expensive. The cost of eight chemotherapy treatments for a single patient can range between $100 and $30,000.[29] When Lynn went on chemo pills after her surgery for kidney cancer, they arrived refrigerated and cost $9,000. **Lynn's husband** commented that *they cost so much they should have been delivered in an armored car.*

Often multiple chemotherapy drugs are used in combination or in sequence, which may increase the costs. In addition, some medications are difficult to obtain early in their life cycles, even though they've been approved for sale by the Food and Drug Administration, because the manufacturer hasn't yet geared up production.

29 *www.livestrong.com.*

When it comes to medication costs, caregivers had very practical suggestions, which included finding out whether reimbursement varies with the prescribed dosage and form of the drug. **Judy T's husband** learned something important about the cost of pharmaceuticals and ways of minimizing insurance co-pays:

> *When Judy started on Procrit, she had 40 units a week in one shot. Then the dosage was increased to 60 units. Our insurance paid 30% for brand name drugs, for a maximum of $100 per month per prescription. If the doctor had prescribed the 60 units in the form of one 40 unit dose and one 20 unit dose, they had different pharmaceutical numbers, so it would have doubled the cost of that drug to us. (It actually cost $3,000 per month at the time, and it costs more now.). So he switched us to three 20s because the three 20s carried the same code number and therefore the same co-pay cost as one 20.*

Caregivers also recommended investigating whether you can qualify for pharmaceutical companies' drug assistance programs. Most pharmaceutical companies have them, and they can serve as resources if you are having difficulty obtaining a medication or need financial assistance to pay for it. After Didier was diagnosed with renal cell carcinoma, **his wife JoAnn** sought a newly approved, hard-to-find, costly medication for his treatment by being resourceful:

> *It's a relatively rare cancer. The medication, Sutent, was hard to get. Also, it cost about $7,500 a month, and insurance would pay 80%. Many drug manufacturers have drug assistance programs, so I called Pfizer. All I had to do was fill out the paperwork, and the drug appeared on my doorstep. I didn't pay anything.*

Programs that offer such assistance can be accessed at the following websites:

- ❧ Partnership for Prescription Assistance, which was created by the pharmaceutical research companies in 2005, catalogs over 475 public and private programs, including nearly 200 provided by pharmaceutical companies. These can be accessed online at *www.pparx.org* or by phone at 1-888-4PPA-NOW.

◊ The Patient Advocate Foundation *(www.patientadvocate. org)*, described above, provides financial assistance with pharmaceutical co-pays for patients who qualify medically and financially.

◊ The American Cancer Society maintains an index of such programs to assist with paying for treatment and managing insurance issues. You can call 800-ACS-2345 or go online to *www.cancer.org* and enter "financial help" or "insurance" in the search engine.

◊ The CancerCare Co-Payment Assistance Foundation has re-designed its website (*www.cancercarecopay.org*) and enriched its offerings. In addition to providing the ability to search the Cancer Financial Assistance Coalition database directly from the website, the foundation provides up to $10,000 per year in co-payment assistance to eligible individuals coping with an assortment of  specific cancer diagnoses, which changes over time as funding sources evolve. The website can provide up-to-date specifics.

Financial concerns—managing complex paperwork, sustaining employment, gaining financial help, and solving insurance problems—loom large and become a primary focus for many cancer caregivers. Sometimes these concerns get overlooked in the flurry of diagnostic and medical issues that arise at the early stages of cancer care. It's important to know ahead of time what to anticipate and what kinds of resources are available to help you through financial, insurance, legal, and employment considerations. Doing so will allow you to take action faster and to minimize associated anxiety, so both you and your patient can concentrate your energies on critically important medical and quality of life issues.

# Chapter Nine

# Seeking Normalcy During Treatment

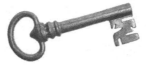

Normalcy for both caregiver and patient disappears quickly after a cancer diagnosis. People who haven't experienced the cancer journey can't imagine how much both patient and caregiver long for the way their life was before cancer. Some say you can get it back; others insist that you can only achieve a "new normal." Of course, there will be times when it feels like cancer has totally taken over all aspects of life, but most of the interviewees tried at least to simulate a sense of normalcy by refusing to define themselves exclusively in terms of the disease.

**Doug's mother** felt it was like the anguish of losing something you valued—life without cancer—no matter how things turn out:

> *A caregiver, like the person with cancer, starts a kind of griev-*
> *ing process from the point of diagnosis. It's like we're grieving*
> *for the loss of "normalcy." Yet we also need to power through*
> *the grief, focus on a cure, and demonstrate hope, so there is*
> *little time to work through the grief.*

Other caregivers felt that, in spite of the life-changing effect of a cancer diagnosis, the quest to recover some form of normalcy is a big part of what their job is all about.

Key topics for exploring this important aspect of caregiving are:

**Creating a Healing Environment**

**Healing Through Humor**

**Letting Help In**

**Relationships with Friends**

## Creating a Healing Environment

Creating a healing environment for someone is a particular challenge when you yourself are feeling anxious and upset, as though your world has been upended. But that is the caregiver's job. It doesn't mean you can't express your emotions—on the contrary, the patient needs to know how much you care about and are committed to his recovery. But the patient also needs you to show a calm demeanor, apply good observation skills and judgment, and partner with him and with the medical team in making life beyond cancer a reality.

### For the Patient

One way to convince the patient that his customary life is still within reach is to treat him normally, to whatever degree possible, even if it's just for part of each day. You want to remind him that:

- He is not his cancer.
- He doesn't need to be defined solely by his cancer.
- His vision of life beyond cancer is worth fighting for.
- He won't be alone throughout the process.

In some ways, **Ellen M's husband** is a model case. He acknowledged what she'd lost when she had brain surgery, and then he set about creating an environment in which she would remember what she still had:

> For someone like Ellen who was very athletic and very independent and loved to drive, taking all of that away from her *[when she lost partial use of her right arm]* was very difficult.

*My main job as a caregiver was to create an environment that was conducive to her recovery.*

*Part of that was encouraging the intellectual stimulation of writing her book during this whole period of time. It was also important for her to find a way to exercise. We laid out a really good regimen she can use in working out about an hour a day. We try to keep her involved with family and sports. She still loves to play golf with one arm.*

*I try to tailor the menu to whatever she's feeling like on a particular day, bring flowers into the house, take her clothes shopping, and make sure she gets a chance to travel to see family and friends. Most of these things would be part of the general maintenance of a relationship. I think when this kind of situation occurs, you have to put all that in hyper drive.*

Some cancer patients are explicit about how they want to be treated, as **Sharon's sister** shared:

*Sharon wanted to be treated the same way as before. "Don't hold back," she said to me when she realized I'd stopped complaining about stupid things like morning traffic. It felt to me like she was sick, so that stuff didn't matter, but she said she'd feel bad if I treated her differently.*

**Michelle's husband**, who also cared for his brother and sister, echoed the same message:

*Treat the patient like you always did. His life has changed. Don't change how you are with him, because there is enough changed in the patient's life already and most other people are treating him differently.*

## For the Caregiver

The message from patients to "treat me like you did before" pertains just as much to caregivers. **Jenn S's husband** found it frustrating that people walked on eggshells around him:

*You don't always need to talk about your feelings; you need to be a normal guy and drink that beer with your friends. Then you go back to work, and everyone knows what's going on, and all you get is those looks. Can somebody just not give me that look? Can you just not work around me today and instead let me do my job? Just treat me like normal.*

For the most part, caregivers felt that even though normalcy had disappeared for them as well as for their patients, they needed to keep their focus on life outside the cancer arena in order to sustain their balance and perspective. **Jen P's husband** explained that:

*Normalcy absolutely* does *exist, even during cancer. Life doesn't stop, the sun doesn't stop rising. The mortgage payment doesn't stop coming around every 30 days. You have to have a life and can't sit around feeling sorry for yourself. That doesn't help you get better. You just have to tough it out.*

One other important thing he realized was that when people treated him normally, he could more easily sustain his ability to treat Jen normally.

For some, like **Amelia's husband**, there were challenges in getting others to treat him as they had in the past:

*A couple of high school friends whom I'd tried to get to visit for years just called and said they were coming. "If you can't see us," they said, "that's fine, but we're coming." It was really comforting, but it was also awkward. It was hard to act normal because everyone was showing so much empathy. I needed normal. I needed to go watch a movie and blank out my mind for a while and have a beer with my friends.*

*One of them, who had become a doctor, wanted to ensure we were getting the right care and asking the right questions. I couldn't see past his focus on being a doctor to find the friend. They were focused on the situation I was in and couldn't give me normal.*

*There's something we call the sad face. You almost have to laugh when people visit you with the sad eyes. You want to say, "Give me a break! Is that all you can do?"*

**Ellsworth's wife** found that the best way to help her husband feel normal while he was dying was to meet one of his unexpected personal requests:

> *One bright spot is that one day he said, "I want you to get in bed with me." It made him feel better, and me, too, because I could hug him.*

There's nothing like a hug to make life feel normal, if only for a few minutes.

## Healing Through Humor

Sometimes it's just stubbornness and dogged perseverance that allow patients and their caregivers to get through the cancer journey with a positive mindset; at other times it's humor. Studies have shown that humor can be therapeutic. Recognized as a complementary therapy by leading health care providers, it is endorsed by many cancer experts, including the American Cancer Society.

While no one claims that humor can cure disease, many studies have shown that it can reduce stress, diminish pain sensations, increase breathing rate and oxygen consumption, and release "feel good" endorphins that boost one's mood. Some sources distinguish between "passive" humor, like watching a funny movie or reading an amusing book, and "spontaneous" humor, which entails recognizing what's comical in day-to-day activities. In the words of comedian Red Skelton, "No matter what your heartache may be, laughing helps you forget it for a few seconds."[30] Or, as **Steve's wife** pointed out, *You need a lot of humor to get through this. The more you laugh, the better you feel.*

Several interviewees actually talked about engaging in spontaneous "black humor" during their treatment periods. When **Jeff's mother** saw her 13-year-old son through aggressive chemotherapy and radiation for Hodgkin's lymphoma, having a sense of humor kept them both going:

> *He lost his hair. He looked so funny. He had hair on the top of his head but not on the lower part. He had sunburn. He*

---

30 *http://izquotes.com/quote/172221.*

*was always laughing and joking about it. At that time, there was a brand of T-shirts and sportswear called "No Fear" that had these really bizarre sayings on them. He wore one every day. That was his motto: "I've got no fear. I'm gonna beat it."*

And so far, eight years later, he has beaten it; and he's still joking.

**Abby**, a minister who was undergoing chemotherapy for ovarian cancer, appreciated her sister's sense of humor:

*Jan saved my hair when it fell out after the first or second treatment. I asked her to shave my head. She did but left me with one bunch at the top. It never fell out. We named it POG. POG stood for "Part of God"—anything that's good. It helped me discover that I could look at myself and not view the cancer as an adversary, but have fun. I never even picked up the wig I had selected. Jan gave me humor nonstop, and I knew I could count on her for the duration.*

Humor strengthened their sisterly bond, and Abby is doing well today.

For **Susan's daughters**, Stacey and Kim, humor at mealtime kept them going. In **Kim's** words:

*We shared lots of humor. Hours and hours worth. Mom was always about food and never lost the need or want for food. Often she'd say she was hungry and forget that I'd fed her a half hour before. She'd come to dinner so happy, like she was going to the White House for dinner. She'd have a huge smile. A couple of nights she looked like she was totally hammered, like Silly Sue came to dinner. Fun, like we were at a party every night, and she'd always loved parties.*

As long as you commit to keep your patient laughing in spite of the cancer and what it might have taken away from him, the journey becomes much more bearable. It might even be filled with amusing and memorable moments.

## Letting Help In

Many of the caregivers said that cancer caregiving isn't a solo job. If you try to do it on your own, you're likely to burn out or simply get overwhelmed by the multiplicity of demands on your time and your energy. Allowing others to help can expand the healing environment and aid in restoring normalcy for everyone involved.

## Building the Team

**Mindy's husband** spoke of the caregiving team from the perspective of a young couple with three young children:

> *You have to create a community of helpers if you don't have one. Pick out the most difficult time of day. For me, it's morning. Getting three kids of different ages ready for school takes two adults. At 6 a.m. every day my mother is here to help. She lives only seven minutes away.*
>
> *Mindy begged me to help keep it as seamless and normal for the kids as we could. Our two moms switched off in the evenings. I didn't need as much help at night, because when she was here, Mindy could do more.*

**Doug's mother** described the need for creating a care team and how it should work:

> *You can't include everyone, so you need to choose your nurturing caregiver group. Decide how much you want from them and what you can give them.*
>
> *The care team is like geese when they're flying in a V formation. They switch off when the leader tires, and another goose takes the lead. So it was with me and my husband. We'd switch off. It was a subtle, nonverbal handoff, but it happened.*

Family members often represent the first go-to option. Susan's daughters divided up caregiving roles almost instinctively, without having to communicate about it. **Stacey** explained how:

> *Early on I stepped out of the knowledge loop of making decisions, and into ways of keeping Mom sane, from being scared. That was my main role. We just knew who was better at what. Kim was better on the Internet, and I was better*

*with the emotional part of it. We're almost like twins. We never discussed it; we just knew. The reliance on each other got us through.*

Sharing responsibilities with the members of one's extended family can be a mixed blessing, however. Whether and how it works out depends on the individuals and the history of family relationships. Some families have trouble reaching an agreement on how to allocate responsibilities and resolve their conflicts during the caregiving process. Different family members cope with stress differently, and depending on their history with the patient, they may have personal issues that can get in the way. The challenge for the primary caregiver is to allow each member to grieve for normalcy in his own way while at the same time ensuring that caregiving needs are met.

The American Society of Clinical Oncologists (ASCO) provides useful information about these kinds of issues. If you're trying to develop a shared caregiving arrangement with other family members or seeking insights about how normal family life and relationships may be affected by cancer, you might find helpful information at *www.cancer.net.*

**Artie's daughter-in-law**, our three-time caregiver, advises that if you don't have a natural family care team, build one by drawing in friends:

*Don't think you're superwoman. Assign help, ask for help. I thought I could do it all with Artie, like having a new baby and sleeping when the baby sleeps. The first time as a caregiver, I wouldn't have recognized the need for help if I'd had a sign in front of my face. Now I say take any help you can get.*

## Learning to Accept Help

For many caregivers, accepting assistance from others beyond their immediate family proved especially challenging. That resistance may stem from embarrassment, or a sense that society expects us to "tough it out alone," or an unwillingness to impose on others. Whatever the reason, your patient needs you to set such personal concerns aside.

Even though **Jenn S's husband** wanted more help, it was also hard for him to let friends in on the "down and dirty" of their family's daily living:

*Everyone wants to help you somehow. Make you dinner, clean your house, do your laundry. Do something. For a while, I felt like we were living in a bed and breakfast because we were coming and going all the time. It takes its toll on you, especially when it becomes a longer process. It was hard to let people help then because our schedules were so unpredictable.*

*Once we got home from the hospital, we were more liberal about letting people come over and clean, or make dinner, or things like that. But no one wants your buddy's wife to see your dirty bathroom. It's one thing to offer help, but they could give you a gift card for a cleaning service. Who cares if Olga sees it? You aren't going to see Olga again.*

In most cases, caregivers indicated that the benefits of allowing others to help by far outweighed any apprehension they might have. **Samantha's mother** says that the first important step is realizing that it's not about trading favors:

*Understand your limitations and that help is a good thing. That person doesn't want you to pay them back. You'll pay them back by helping someone else.*

*Some people just gave things without asking. When people did ask, I realized it was stupid not to acknowledge our needs since I knew these people well. I learned it was way too big, bigger than me and bigger than Sam, for me to think I was equipped to do this alone. It was kind of the "it takes a village" idea.*

**Joe's wife** acknowledges that letting others help took time, but she now realizes that letting them in was not only important support for her and her family, but was also a gift to those who offered the help:

*I'm trying to get better at letting other people help us. I'm really trying as I get older, because I realize it makes me feel good when someone trusts me with something to do for them, so I'm starting to realize they're really serious when they offer to help me. Some people come in and offer to cure world hunger for you, and that's just talk. But I could believe someone who says, "If you'll go home and take a shower, I'll stay here, and you can be back in an hour, and I won't leave this room," because it was specific and I knew they'd be there.*

**Ellen W's husband** is another caregiver who is still finding it hard to accept as much help as their large network of friends is ready to give, even though he realizes that some feel bad when they're not allowed to help. In many cases, caregivers are reluctant because they don't know what to say when friends ask, "How can I help?" or "What can I do to help?" Having to deal with an open-ended question, making yet another decision when they are already overwhelmed, feels like the last straw. As **Paul's wife** explained:

*In retrospect, I can appreciate that everyone asks how they can help, but I appreciate it more when they give me choices. The things you really need are to make a meal, clean the house, do laundry or shopping—not just open-ended offers.*

**Doug's mother** agreed and echoed that sentiment:

*You crave being normal, and that's hard for anyone to give you. One thing that really helped was that someone cared for our lawn. I wouldn't have thought to ask. So if you're offering help, the best thing to do is to say, "I'd like to do this. Is that OK?" Don't ask an open-ended question.*

Similarly, the people who helped **Joe's wife**, who didn't have the energy to make additional decisions during Joe's treatment, came to her aid in a way that worked well:

*The people who it was easier to let help were the ones who just did it. Some friends called the kids and said, "We're bringing dinner over tonight." It was a done deal. No one had to feel obligated. It didn't force me to make a decision.*

*I had a friend from out of town who sent Omaha steaks that could just be cooked in the oven or frozen foods that the kids could fix for themselves. It was a no-brainer, and I*

*was grateful because I didn't want to have to decide what I
needed them to do. You're so tired that after a while, you can
hardly form a plan.*

## Facilitating Help from Others

Despite their best intentions, friends and associates may benefit from
some guidance. If you're a caregiver and someone asks that terrible open-
ended question about what help you could use, think beyond food. Consider letting someone take out the trash, do the food shopping, drive the kids
to their weekend activities, or provide a gift certificate for a house cleaning from a local service. Then there's always cutting the lawn, plowing or
shoveling the snow, or even weeding the garden for someone who takes
particular pride in his yard and doesn't have the time or energy to keep up
with it. Finally, think about whether you and your patient might benefit
from a night off by having someone take the kids for a movie or overnight,
or maybe having someone accompany your patient to his several-hour chemotherapy infusion so you'd have some time off.

**Paul's wife** had some suggestions for new caregivers:

*When people ask how they can help, don't be afraid to ask for
basic things. People want to help but don't know how. Give
a list to your best friend and ask her to work it through with
those who want to help.*

For **Tim S's wife**, it was clearer what she *didn't* need than what
she did:

*My daughters made a list of things that people could do if
they wanted to help if they were here. It included fixing food,
reading to Dad, things my mom likes to do, and so on. Some
of them were just daily living kinds of things.*

Her notion of having a list of responsibilities that others can take off
your shoulders bears underscoring. Taking the time to put together such
a list will make it much easier for you to "cope" with requests from others
who want to help.

**Artie's daughter-in-law** had great suggestions on this topic:

᷒ Keep a cooler with ice in it outside the front door so people can bring meals at their convenience and not have to worry about coordinating a drop-off time with you.

᷒ Ask them to leave instructions as to how to warm the food.

᷒ Keep a basket of Hershey's Kisses by the door in little fabric bags with thank-you notes attached. This will keep you from having to do individual "thank yous" for people who help out.

᷒ Keep a spreadsheet of what people have brought you and whether they've been thanked and when.

The bottom line is: Don't hesitate to say "no" if an offer of help is made at a difficult time for you, but remember that the more you let others help, the better they'll get at understanding *how* to help.

## Relationships with Friends

Friends can help patients and caregivers strive for normalcy whether they are close by or far away. Even a brief visit or occasional phone call can break the sense of isolation that often descends during the cancer journey. It's important to recognize the value of such casual encounters and acknowledge their benefit, especially for people who would like to be more involved but can't be for a variety of reasons.

### Friends as Part of the Support Team

For **Tim S's wife**, friends who lived at a distance were immensely helpful in the overall support process. Although they couldn't be there often or offer tangible day-to-day support, their sustained relationships over time were nourishing in their own way:

> We had a very good friend in Michigan whom we'd seen about once a year in the past. The night of Tim's MRI, I had gotten a letter from her. She was among the first people we

*had called, and she wrote me every week thereafter. She came
to visit a couple of times. It was a long-distance relationship
that intensified over this period.*

**Claire's daughter** felt enriched by the support that her mother's
childhood friends provided to Claire during the cancer treatment:

*She had two best friends from the sixth grade. They did a
lot for her. They took her to appointments and pretty much
went to sit with her every day. One of them I now see as
much as I can. She's like my mother now, and I talk with her
all the time.*

Many caregivers said they had both positive and negative surprises
when it came to friends who offered help and support. **Debbie B's husband** explained that people they expected would help sometimes didn't,
while others offered unexpected acts of kindness:

*Some people dive in and surprise you. Debbie had a small
number of very close friends. One of the people outside of
this small group offered to come with her when she was having chemo. She's one of a couple of people who really came
out of the woodwork and were there for Debbie. Her best
friend still sends me an email almost every morning.*

The support from her felt totally normal because it was an extension of
their past friendship.

Finally, there are the friends who bond so tightly that they sustain their
normal friendship to keep the patient from losing heart during treatment.
**Robbi's friend** (who is herself a long-time breast cancer survivor) was
determined not to let Robbi go through treatment alone:

*Robbi was a stage IV ovarian cancer patient. Six friends and
I created a Chemo Club. We'd go to chemo with her and play
cards and games. We were all there together maintaining our
normal chatter. It created positive memories. As caregivers,
we were a group of friends who wanted to help by acting on
that friendship.*

The support experience reinforced their camaraderie and sent an important message to each of them that if they were ever diagnosed with cancer, they wouldn't have to go through it alone.

Judy M's friends provided a similar psychological and social safety net, allowing **Judy** to express her deepest concerns:

> *My women friends spontaneously offered help. They kept the mood upbeat, and there was lots of laughing. I shared with them that I was afraid I wouldn't make it. I never said it to my husband because I don't think we could have faced it. That was the only time I shared my fear.*

We should all have such friends.

## Pull-Aways

On the other hand, some caregivers experienced "pull-aways"—formerly close friends or family members who literally withdrew when the going got tough and a cancer diagnosis tested their loyalty and commitment. That's a blow to feelings of normalcy, and it is particularly hurtful to the patient at a time when he needs old friends and relatives more than ever.

Many caregivers and their patients were philosophical about pull-aways. **Michelle's husband** explained that this phenomenon is something that caregivers should expect:

> *The cancer patient is part of a club that no one wants to join. Most people don't know how to deal with the cancer patient or their family. They pull away. It's not that they don't care, but they will ask other people how the patient is doing, and they won't call directly. Seven out of 10 people are like that, in that they don't know what to say. Cancer is everyone's biggest fear.*

**Carole's husband** had prior experience with cancer. He offered a similar explanation:

> *My youngest brother died of cancer at age 17. Many of his friends pulled away because they couldn't deal with their own mortality issues.*

It is just as difficult when a sibling, intimate friend, or lover pulls away. This happened to **Barbara** when her boyfriend said he couldn't handle her having breast cancer. Similarly, Tahira's boyfriend broke off their relationship shortly after her breast cancer diagnosis. As **Tahira's mother** explained:

> *Tahira had been in a semi-serious relationship when she started chemo, and he walked. He was a very tight person, obsessed with perfection. This was disorderly, and he couldn't handle it. I was the first to hold the door for him as he left.*

Fortunately, both of these young women were strong enough fighters to get through their cancers without letting the pull-away of their significant others upset them enough to slow their recovery.

## Sustaining Normal Social Relationships

Another aspect of creating a sense of normalcy has to do with helping cancer patients and their caregivers sustain social relationships so they can have a life outside of their cancer experience. **James' wife** found that friends' efforts to spend time with her outside of a hospital setting were important ways to keep her connected with life beyond caring for James:

> *If you can, find time to grab a cup of coffee together or pull the caregiver offline to get out of the hospital environment and to talk about other things.*

Some caregivers, like **Jacqueline's husband**, took the initiative to invite others into their homes to sustain interactions:

> *There wasn't anything others could do, except drop by and be friendly and have a drink, just like before. Friends didn't shy away. I realized the process wouldn't be that long. You don't want to be like a leper, so the house was always open. Sometimes when she was going through the chemo, she'd come down in a long beautiful gown with a bandana around her head looking very attractive.*

**Mike S's wife** says it was an adaptive strategy to have friends come visit them:

> *Since we couldn't join our wonderful friends in going out, we'd ask them to drop by for a glass of wine. It lessened our feeling of isolation. A few pulled away, but I didn't have the emotional energy to care at the time.*

Sustaining normal relationships is essential to healing, within reason. For **Tim S's wife**, these kinds of gatherings were helpful up to a point. She realizes she didn't have people visit as often as she might have, but sometimes people who did visit stayed too long:

> *When people were here, conversations were good and there were lots of good remembrances. There were also several times when people were here that Tim said he'd like people to go home.*

Normalcy is precious. Most of us don't fully appreciate it until it's gone. Hopefully the ideas from other caregivers that were shared in this chapter will give you a sense of how to move toward normalcy as you work through the cancer experience. The closer you can get, the more you'll be helping your patient heal and overcome the sense of isolation, uncertainty, and fear that could be just around the next corner.

# Chapter Ten

# Children and Cancer

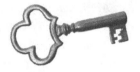

Children are supposed to be carefree, with lots of time for playing, learning, building friendships, and growing physically and emotionally. They're supposed to have their whole lives ahead of them. They're not supposed to get life-threatening illnesses. When the word "cancer" enters their world, caregivers naturally experience strong reactions, regardless of whether the child is the patient or is part of a household that's immersed in a cancer battle.

This chapter shares some compelling stories from parents who have experienced the emotional roller coaster that's involved in helping children to cope with cancer. They are organized against four topics::

> **When the Patient is a Child**
>
> **When There's Cancer in the Family**
>
> **When Children Lose a Parent to Cancer**
>
> **Resources for Caregivers Concerned About Children**

## When the Patient is a Child

It shouldn't come as a surprise that a cancer diagnosis for a child puts parents through an emotional wringer. After all, aren't they supposed to protect their kids? Aren't they supposed to be able to explain unexpected or uncomfortable events and make them go away? Almost all of the parental caregivers described how a child's serious cancer diagnosis provoked such intense feelings of profound helplessness, it was hard to maintain the focus, stability, and calm required to make rational caregiving decisions and to advocate effectively with medical providers.

**Jeff's mother** explained what it was like to see him going through cancer treatment for stage IVA Hodgkins disease when he was only 13 years old:

> *It was devastating. I was in denial and angry. What do you say when your kid asks, "Mommy, am I going to die?" How do you say you don't know? I remember him lying in the bed and just screaming because he was in such pain. You can't make it go away, you can't make it better. You're supposed to kiss the booboo and make it all go away. You'd trade places with him a million times over if you could, because you don't want to see your kid go through that kind of pain.*

**Doug's mother** had a similar experience when her 14-year-old son was being treated for Ewing's sarcoma:

> *When the medical team members were hurting him, I didn't know what to do. It made me feel helpless, but I didn't want to do more harm through my reaction. If his oncologist hadn't come in right then, I don't know what I'd have done. Observing it, we concluded we'd never EVER leave him by himself again. There were times when things were more predictable and you knew the staff on duty, but every time there could be an OMIGOD moment, we made sure we were present. It was a great comfort to him to know that someone was there.*

You might be wondering why I'm emphasizing this point. After all, who wouldn't be emotional in caring for a child battling cancer? The problem is that some parents let their emotions hijack their minds when they're interacting with the medical team. They may be angry and agitated, which in turn may lead them to take their frustration out on the physicians and other team members when treatments cause the child any level of avoidable discomfort.

This is what happened with **Lanie's mother**, and it prevented her from communicating as an effective advocate. When Lanie, age nine, was having sustained headaches and started vomiting for no explainable reason, her mother pressed the doctor for a clear diagnosis. But getting that clarity took several months and trips to different medical providers. Her pediatrician originally attributed the symptoms to lactose intolerance or to her mother's "strong personality." Finally, a specialized children's hospital determined that Lanie had a rare pilocytic astrocytoma tumor of the cerebellum, one so rare that there was only one other child in the world with the same tumor at the time.

In hindsight, it's possible that the medical team may never have explained the situation clearly—how large the tumor was, where it was, and how it might spread into Lanie's spine and kill her—but it's also possible that Lanie's mother couldn't hear what was being said. She was desperate to save her daughter and to reduce Lanie's pain and suffering. She was an active advocate but felt that requests to minimize Lanie's pain were ignored. As Lanie's condition worsened, her mother became so aggressive toward the medical team that she was nearly thrown out of the hospital. Lanie died 11 months after her diagnosis, having suffered significant pain and paralysis.

Lanie's mother remains angry to this day. By the time I interviewed her, it was 16 years later. At first, she seemed like a strong and reasonable person, but when she started to talk about how she felt the medical system had wronged her, she underwent a complete transformation: She started to rant and rave, got red in the face, began gesturing aggressively, and paced back and forth like someone possessed. In light of her story, it was easy to imagine that such behavior might have offended and alienated the medical professionals charged with saving Lanie's life.

Unfortunately, a social worker or clinical psychologist didn't enter the scene soon enough to ease the situation. In fact, when a psychiatrist was brought in, he ended up as the advocate for the hospital, rather than serving as a mediator to build mutual understanding. In retrospect, it's difficult to tell whether there were times when more compassion and more reasoned judgment on both sides might have made both Lanie and her mother more comfortable, or what might have happened differently if her mother had been a calmer, more composed advocate.

In contrast, **Samantha's mother** had a calm style and collaborative approach. It probably also helped that she was consulting with hospital organizations and knew a lot about doctors when two-year-old Samantha was diagnosed with leukemia:

> *Having been in health care and knowing my daughter was so young that I'd need to be an advocate, I was determined to learn everything I could so I'd understand what was going on, could interpret the decisions her doctors were making, and could be part of the process. Fortunately, the pediatric intensive care doctor whom we first saw in the emergency room viewed the relationship with the caregiver as a partnership, so he would tell me what they were going to do in advance and go over the care plan to make sure I was in the loop.*
>
> *In the hospital, I was determined that I needed to know that the time there was being well used and that Samantha was being protected from infections by being kept there as short a time as possible. When I saw inefficiencies, I requested a meeting with the head nurse and whomever else she wanted to bring. I asked them to take a half-day out of the routine three-day in-hospital treatment cycle. All I knew was that I had to protect Sam. I thought they'd say I was the mother from hell, but I didn't care.*
>
> *Instead of being angry or challenging me, they took everything down that I said and thanked me for taking the initiative. They made sure we had nurses that we had worked with before and would focus on us and be as efficient as they could.*

At one point, her non-confrontational style allowed Sam's mother to convey information between nursing teams to enhance two-year-old Samantha's tolerance for her therapy:

> *I had heard from the outpatient nurses that if you reversed the order in which the drugs were delivered, the patient would*

*do better and have a less negative physical reaction. So when I saw the hospital nurses doing it the old way, I asked them to stop and told them about the alternative sequence.*

*They said they didn't know about it, so I asked them to call the outpatient nurse and ask. The outpatient team came to the floor to review the process with Sam's nursing team. Her nurses switched the order of the infusions; Sam reacted well, and the team realized that I'd been right.*

Once again, the bottom line on being an advocate is that if your gut tells you something isn't right, ask the professional caregivers to explain what they are doing and why, and to change it if necessary. If their answer isn't satisfactory to you, ask to see the supervising nurse or doctor. It's perfectly acceptable for you to do so and to work your way up the chain of command. Just be aware that your understandable concerns may prove counterproductive if you let them make you too intense and emotional to collaborate with the medical team.

### Restoring the Child's Social Environment

Children with cancer often experience unique issues regarding their social relationships. It's particularly hard for a parent to see his child's friends disappear because the friends don't understand their own fear and discomfort with the emotions surrounding cancer. **Michael S's father** saw that happen with his son:

*Michael had been a good-looking kid and a star in the actors guild at school, but after his surgery he looked like a refugee from a Frankenstein movie. He had three friends who stuck by him and became life-long friends. They stuck by him even when he was in the hospital, and they made sure he got to the senior prom.*

*A huge other group who were supposedly his friends fell away. We noticed it, too, with our friends. People who aren't used to personal crises back away and don't know how to deal with you.*

Understanding pull-aways is harder for a child—especially a child with cancer.

**Doug's mother** realized early on in his treatment that her son was having trouble staying in touch with the aspects of his high school experience that had once defined his normal life:

> *Doug recovered from surgery without complications and resumed rigorous chemo. The medical team thought it better if he not return to school for his sophomore year, so we had him tutored at home. He missed his sports and friends, and he felt cut off. We saw signs that Doug was getting depressed. He craved normalcy, but it was out of reach. His life had been totally upended. So I helped him to re-establish his connections.*

His mom's outreach was so successful that during Doug's last days three years later, his friends attended his brother's eighth-grade graduation in Doug's place and were at Doug's bedside when he died.

## When the Child's Diagnosis is Grim

Children aren't supposed to die, but the harsh truth of cancer is it that doesn't obey any rules about what's rational or fair. When a child is seriously ill and at risk of dying, you need particularly effective and sensitive guidance. An excellent resource is the booklet, "What Do We Do Now?," by Quality of Life Publishing (QoL). It provides an overview of how to handle the key issues, as well as offering a list of other reference resources on the topic. In general the content parallels the ideas and examples offered in this book, but with a special focus on the age of the patient. Most of QoL's publications are made available to institutions in the form of "branded" booklets, but you can access a single copy by calling 877-513-0099 or going online to *www.QoLpublishing.com.*

## Helping Children Cope with Survivor Guilt

When the news is good and a child is cured of cancer, parents' challenges may not be over. Jeff overcame his childhood Hodgkin's lymphoma. Yet one of the most impactful experiences for **Jeff's mother**, in the aftermath of his "re-birthday" bone marrow transplant, was seeing how Jeff reacted to learning that other children whom he had befriended during his treatment didn't survive their cancers:

> *I remember Jeff sitting on the kitchen floor sobbing as he asked, "Mom, why not me?" One of the hardest things for me was when Jeff was leaving the hospital, after his transplant. One of his friends, a boy his same age, had leukemia and was terminal. It tore me up to say good-bye to this friend and his mother when I knew I was taking my son home and he was going to be fine, but this boy wouldn't.*

Cancer isn't a rational disease. There's often no clear reason why one patient makes it through and another dies. Rather than trying to explain it to a child experiencing survivor guilt, all you can do is express your relief that your child was one of the lucky ones.

## Helping Healthy Siblings Avoid Feelings of Neglect

When one child in a family has cancer, the other siblings may need special attention. Caregivers say that it's too easy to focus all of your waking energy on the sick child. Depending on their age, engaging healthy siblings in caring for the one who has cancer can help to both manage their expectations and let them know how much you love and trust them. Even though daily life has been severely disrupted, it's important to sustain routines that will help the healthy siblings to preserve whatever remnants of normalcy they can.

**Jeff's mother** still remembers that early on in his treatment for Hodgkin's lymphoma, she got an earful from his sister:

> *One day my daughter, who was 16, asked, "Mom, do I have to get sick too to get your attention? Because I'm not here anymore." It was like all of a sudden you see the light. You're so focused on the child who is sick, I don't know how families who have more than one child do it. You say to yourself, "Whoa! Thank God she was in tune enough with her feelings to say it." She did both of us a favor. She helped me realize that I needed to pay more attention to her needs too.*

*After that, we set aside one night a week to do something together, even though Jeff was hospitalized or recovering at home. We'd go to a movie, shopping, or out with her friends. We left her father in charge of her brother.*

In the case of one blended family, four-year-old **Michael L's mother** focused right away on bringing the other children into the process of caring for him:

*Jack and I had been planning our marriage at the time Michael was diagnosed. We'd already blended our families for two years—his three children and my Michael. Michael was 4, and the other boys were 9, 12, and 13. Even though we were close already, we became even closer through Michael's cancer journey.*

*For 12 weeks, every day Jack would get the kids to school and pick them up, and then they'd all come to the hospital to have dinner. The staff and the social workers really catered to our needs. They always had ways to keep the other boys involved and interested, feeling like everyone cared about them too.*

*When it was time for Michael to go home, I became germophobic and had the kids change their clothes when they got back from school and wash their hands and arms up to their elbows. We converted the playroom into a cozy bedroom so Michael could rest and play in the same place.*

*Justin became a caretaker at age 9. He kept a notebook and called himself Dr. Albert. When he and Michael played, Justin would track Michael's food and liquid intake.*

*It's changed the family in a good way. Right after Jack and I got married, we piled the six of us into the car and spent our honeymoon at Camp Sunshine.[31] We'd all been through so much turmoil together, now we needed to have fun together.*

---

31  Camp Sunshine *(www.campsunshine.org)* is a free camp in Maine for children with life-threatening illnesses, together with their families. According to the website, "The year-round program is free of charge to all families and includes 24-hour onsite medical and psychosocial support."

By paying attention to the other children in the household, Michael's mother managed to make caring for him a family activity that actually enriched every member's experience.

## When There's Cancer in the Family

When you have children and there's cancer in the family or a cancer patient in the house, you may feel torn between being honest and worrying that you'll upset or scare them. This section deals with:

- ✌ Telling the Children
- ✌ The Healing (and Distracting) Impact of Children
- ✌ Letting Children Ease the Patient's Dying Process
- ✌ Dealing with Death and Grief

Each of these topics is useful in itself, but the combination will build your confidence in helping children learn how to deal with seriously ill family members.

### Telling the Children

Determining what to say to children when a parent, sibling, or close relative has cancer is always a sensitive decision because you're trying to explain that things are different while at the same time trying not to scare them. Caregivers who shared such stories tended to adjust the message to the age of the child and the severity of the diagnosis. They all recommended telling the truth, managing children's expectations so they can prepare themselves for what's to come, and engaging them to keep the patient company so they can express their affection and maintain as much normalcy in their interactions as possible.

Because younger children are naturally curious, they often observe that something has changed even before they are told. Caregivers who dealt with such children felt it was important at least to acknowledge the new reality, so that it would be OK for the children to ask questions.

161

When Tim N was diagnosed with cancer at age 42, his children were ages 9 and 12. **Tim N's wife** commented that:

> Being honest is the only way you can go when you have kids and are faced with cancer, because the kids know what's going on. They didn't even need to overhear something. I'm sure with the phone conversations going on and everyone's dire looks, they knew something was up. To know what it was, they needed some sort of tangible boundaries put on the thing so they could understand it and put it in its place.
>
> After the pathology came back, I returned home after being at the hospital all day. The kids had been sleeping with me every night. They got in bed with me and asked, "How's Daddy?" I said, "He's OK and will be home in a few more days, but you guys can come in and see him."
>
> Then one of them asked me if he had cancer. I was going to tell them that night anyway, but one of them beat me to it. I told them everything the doctors had been telling us. "They think they got it all, and there wasn't any cancer anywhere else and nothing in the lymph nodes, so it was really good news. And he'll be home really soon."
>
> They didn't ask whether he would die, because it looked like he would be OK. They were really frightened, but Tim and I had always been extremely honest with the kids, age-appropriate.

Rob, age 29, was in the midst of a chondroid chordoma diagnosis during the ramp-up to Christmas. He knew that his children had observed the flurry of unusual activity and suspected that it wasn't holiday-related. **Rob's wife** described how they handled it:

> I didn't want to tell them anything, but they could sense that something was different because I was on the computer all the time. The night before the biopsy, we had to tell the kids something. So I just said, "Daddy has something in his head that doesn't belong there. The doctors are going to take a look and figure out what it is. When he gets home, he'll be tired,

*but he will still be your same dad." One of them asked, "Is Daddy going to die?"*

*We had agreed ahead of time that we had to be honest, so I told them that as soon as we knew more, we'd tell them more. For three months before surgery, we never used the word "cancer" in conversation with our kids. That's a word that scares kids.*

Dealing with the unknown can be the most difficult aspect for younger children. It helped Ellen W's eight-year-old daughter to meet the hospital social worker and to see where her mom was receiving chemotherapy. **Ellen W's husband** explained that:

*We keep it as light as we can. "Mom's going to the hospital." Our daughter knows it's cancer but we tell her that the doctors are doing all the right stuff to make mommy better. No odds or anything. We brought her in to watch Ellen get chemo, and our social worker took her around and gave her a tour of the medical oncologist's office area, so he and she are buddies now.*

*One day I took her to the museum nearby while Ellen was getting treated. Frankly, our daughter finds it all a little boring.*

Ellen and her husband engaged their daughter in ways that let her see where her mother was going so often. Just the fact that she finds it boring demonstrates that they've managed to minimize the sense of drama that they were experiencing.

Mindy and her husband were challenged by the age spread of their children and the fact that they would need to communicate differently with each of them about the situation. They hadn't solved the issue completely, but they were making meaningful progress. **Mindy's husband** explained that after they received the diagnosis of metastatic melanoma in Mindy's brain:

*Our son and our older daughter have been awesome. They've protected their little sister so she doesn't know. Our son doesn't show his emotions much. Our older daughter runs through the whole gamut of emotions. Our toddler just laughs and brings all of us joy because she doesn't know. We all envy that.*

*I had to have a heart to heart, brutally honest talk with our older daughter when she was 8. I said, "You've got to understand that things won't be as you want them ever again. It won't get better later." It was a hard lesson.*

*I felt guilty of robbing them of part of their carefree-ness during their childhood. Our older daughter doesn't smile as much as she used to. She's very verbal and plays that she's the oncologist for her stuffed animals. It's her way of putting herself in control. I'm still concerned about our son's lack of openness in talking about how he feels.*

All of these parents had a loving but direct approach to sharing the hardest message of their lives with their young children.

Older children often pose even more of a challenge than younger ones. Little children often guide you with the questions they ask; they let you know how much they are ready to hear. Older children may profess to want total truth but aren't always ready to hear it, so their parents can help them by minimizing the resulting disruption in their lives. There are no easy answers about how to reach a good balance.

In general, as with younger children, caregivers told their older children the truth but adjusted the message to the severity of the diagnosis. The most difficult challenge was managing older children's expectations in situations where the outcome was unknown because they are able to project alternative outcomes.

When James was diagnosed with incurable multiple myeloma, he and his wife decided not to tell their children, who were in the same college, until a pre-scheduled parents' weekend five weeks later. **James' wife** explained:

*We wanted to tell them in person. It's hard to tell your kids that their father has incurable cancer. We had discussed it and didn't want the kids feeling they needed to come home every weekend. So we decided to tell them the good, bad, and ugly so they wouldn't worry that things were being hidden or held back.*

*We kept to that game plan. They asked what the doctor had said, and we said he'd have two to three years with standard treatments, but we've learned about new stuff, especially bone marrow transplants, that could make it better. Information was a tool for them as well. The kids were comforted by knowing that we'd told them everything.*

That was over 24 years ago. As of this writing, James continues to do well.

Some caregivers limited the information shared with their post college-age children to the point where the parent's death came as a shock to them. That's what happened when **Lynn's husband** followed the wishes of his wife to manage the flow of information to their children and keep the news cheerful. When she died, they were in shock because they had had so little warning:

*Our son was in Manhattan, and our daughter in Belgium. She was finishing her master's degree there, and it was Lynn's preference for her not to keep running home. We gave them thumbnails which were always positive and hopeful. In fact, things were upbeat until three days before she died. After the funeral, our daughter was upset and said, "You didn't tell me the truth!"*

He, too, had been stunned by how quickly the situation turned from positive to terminal, but it was hard for their daughter to accept. In the end, there's no easy answer about how to handle such a situation, except to say that this type of no-win dilemma often arises. Sometimes the healthy parent will need to think it through and decide that doing something other than what the patient requested is the best solution for the child's future emotional well-being. All the healthy parent can do is make the best possible decision under the circumstances, showing love to all concerned but with eyes open to the potential negative consequences. Then be prepared to work through them after the fact.

**Annie's husband** had just as challenging a circumstance in informing their adult children about her condition:

> *How do you tell your adult kids that their mother is dying? Explaining to them so they'd comprehend was hard. I could see that a couple of our boys didn't understand why she had all the surgeries or that she was dying. The two girls—one is a cardiac nurse and the other a clinical psychologist—knew what was going on and understood.*
>
> *You don't want to shove it down their throats, but you want them to be aware that things are happening that they're not privy to, and there could be dire results. It was hard for a couple of them in the aftermath.*

Life is about making choices, and in an unpredictable serious cancer situation, there are no easy ones as far as managing the information flow to children is concerned.

## The Healing (and Distracting) Impact of Children

Children can bring joy in many ways. Most of us have experienced how a child's giggle can make us laugh, or how a hug or an adoring look can warm our hearts. One of the great things about children is that they lack the self-consciousness that sometimes causes adults to pull away from a cancer patient. For kids, you are who you are, even if you don't have hair, or are on oxygen, or are feeling queasy. The impact of a child's presence can be great for a cancer patient.

Some caregivers told wonderful stories about how children had had a soothing impact on cancer patients just by being themselves. When Susan was diagnosed with a terminal brain tumor, her daughter Stacey was pregnant, and Susan was given the opportunity to interact with the baby right after he was born. **Stacey's sister Kim** explained that:

> *Stacey had labor induced so Mom could be there at the birth. They put her in a chair that was convertible to a bed. When she'd get tired, she'd lie down next to Stacey. We put her in a wheelchair when Stacey gave birth. She was the*

*first to hold the baby. He was a little bundle of joy for her. We'd wrap him up and she would hold him in bed. We'd joke that it was her turn to watch him. So she was a part of it. It brought a sense of normalcy. He was her first grandson after having had four granddaughters.*

**Mike S's wife** still remembers how their first grandchild, who was born shortly before he got sick, allowed for some warm family moments to distract from his medical situation during his treatment.

*Anne saw to it that our granddaughter visited every day at the house or the hospital. One day, Mike had a minor procedure and Anne brought Isabel right into the recovery room and plunked her down on Mike's chest. When the nurse came in to take his vital signs and everything was normal, she said, "I can tell what kind of medication Mike needs."*

Some families found the daily routine to be a welcome distraction from their total focus on the patient's cancer. **Jen P's husband** explained that:

*We had little kids who needed what little kids need, and we didn't have time to sit around and mope and feel sorry for ourselves because day-to-day life things didn't stop for us. Diapers and naps. They needed us. It was helpful—it forced us to take our minds off ourselves because there were others depending on us for their lives.*

**Mike S's wife** said that Mike found the active involvement of their older children in his care enriched and greatly improved the quality of his life:

*Each of our three children played a significant role in caregiving. They put their own lives on hold to place Mike first. It was impressive and inspiring. I think when Mike would announce, contrary to all evidence, that he was the luckiest man alive, he was marveling in being able to witness the unselfishness of his young adult children. One day, I asked our daughter if spending so much time with us was putting a strain on her family. Her answer was, "In a perfect world, we wouldn't be here so much, but it's not a perfect world."*

*Our son Josh was a wonderful cook. Josh would cook things he thought might appeal to Mike. Josh was never discouraged when Mike ate only a spoonful. Josh also participated in the direct caregiving, initially just as a companion. Later, Josh picked up nursing skills, helping Mike with dressing, hydration, and so on. I think the physical touching involved in helping his father do daily things was important. Men and male children are less likely to touch each other or to hug.*

*Our other son, Jonah, would settle in with Mike to watch sports in the evening, though neither of them was a particularly avid sport fan. Mike could be on the couch and doze off. When he woke up, Jonah would give him the score and an update. It gave them time together doing something they wouldn't ordinarily have done.*

*Jonah would declare cancer-free weekends. He'd rent a van and we would go to a local inn or on a field trip to some place happy and fun. I thought it was brilliant. It was restorative for all of us. We all saw each other daily. We all knew the prognosis right from the start, so we knew that every day we had together was a day more than we could expect.*

## Letting Children Ease the Patient's Dying Process

Children take their lead from their parents about handling and preparing for a loved one's death. To the degree that you can encourage them to ask questions and to interact with the patient during his decline, they will be left with far less unfinished business. They are likely to ask questions even if they aren't told explicitly what is happening, so it may be useful to decide when and how to share information, rather than waiting to react to questions that might arise at awkward times.

**Artie's daughter-in-law** had the most extensive and sensitive story about coaching her children (ages eight and five) through Artie's dying process. Her approach in helping them deal with the pending death of their grandfather, who was living in the house, offers helpful lessons for any of us who may face that situation:

*We were completely honest with our kids, age appropriate-ly. We'd try to screen it. My dad had been through a bout of lung cancer before this, so they weren't strangers to the word "cancer."*

*We set up hospice way before we needed it. The woman from hospice would come and do arts and crafts with the kids, what she called "heart play." They talked about how Papa was dying, and she suggested a wonderful thing for them to do. She asked, "Do you want to make a memory box and windmill, so every time you see it blow, you can think that's Papa with you?" She was laying the groundwork for the healing process afterward.*

*I had been so nervous about the kids, but we had them come in while he was dying to give Artie hugs and kisses. They said their good-byes. It was tremendously stressful, but having him die at home was the most rewarding thing we could have done.*

*The night after he died, I thought I was going to have a problem getting our son back into his room, so we offered to move his own bed back in there right away, but they both climbed into the hospital bed and went to sleep. They still have a pillowcase that they call "Papa's pillowcase," and they have it in a baggie so it still smells like Papa. They still fight over who gets to sleep with Papa. They came up with that themselves.*

*The woman from hospice came back three or four times after Artie died. They filled the memory box right after and put the windmill on the mailbox. The memory box says "I love Papa" on it. It's filled with little things: One of his mints, his watch, his wallet—just little things.*

*I was most worried and concerned about helping the kids get through this. I figured that if I'm stressed, they've gotta be stressed. There were times when they would totally act out because they wanted more attention. They struggled through it too, but it was what was right for us.*

For this family, and for many others, being open with the kids allowed the children to enrich the patient's dying moments and to sustain positive memories that helped everyone in the household.

## When Children Lose a Parent to Cancer

One of the hardest caregiver challenges arises when the patient is one of the children's parents. In the late stages of his life, **Tim N's wife** tried to ensure that his death would not be more devastating than necessary for their children:

> We had to be ready because we had to go on. There's a point where it's almost not about the person who dies. It's more about what will make it OK for the ones who live.
>
> It doesn't mean you have to tell the kids he's going to die, but you have to say, "He's really sick and having lots of problems right now, and his heart is really weak." At that point they might ask, "Is he going to die?" and I'd say, "I hope not, but it's possible. He could die." That was really important for the kids to hear.
>
> In fact, that's how it played out. It was a way of being honest with them and making them feel a part of it. Kids know what's going on. They really do. It's way worse to let a child imagine whatever his mind is going to conjure up rather than tell him concretely and tangibly what's happening, so he doesn't have to worry or feel like you've lied to him and he can't trust what you're saying.

She continued to explain that her children have had a difficult time in the period since Tim died:

> The kids were 12 and 15 when he died, and they're 16 and 19 now. Helping them through it was and continues to be really difficult. I am very open and honest with the kids because trust is the most important thing. When he died, I was numb. Then I started to cry all the time, loudly. The kids understood that I grieved.

*They grieved too. My younger one had her therapist to help. My older daughter didn't start to grieve until this past summer, after she got out of high school. She wanted to be like every other normal kid and didn't tell anyone. She didn't want to be different, to be the kid whose father had died. Both of them put how they really felt about it on hold for a while.*

*It wasn't easy. You just put one foot ahead of the other and try to make the right decisions every day with your kids and yourself. It still isn't easy. My entire life is completely different and will never ever be the same.*

In many cases, when a child's feelings about the death of a parent aren't dealt with candidly, they may not surface until many years later. **Margaret and Bill's son** lost both of his parents to cancer, his 45-year-old mother when he was in high school and his father four years later. In fact, he didn't even learn that she had been treated for cervical cancer until he read it on her death certificate years later. He never had the opportunity to confront his own grief until he helped a friend whose father was dying:

*I relived the death of both of my parents through a friend, whose father was diagnosed with leukemia. He was devastated. I was going to the hospital or staying with him at the house every few days for nearly nine months. I sat with his dad when he was on a respirator. I relived and felt for the first time what it was like to be a caregiver.*

*My friend expressing his raw emotions was the total opposite of the way I had motored on. I needed that. It helped me let my emotions out. Now I'm not ashamed of crying. I suppressed so much when my mother died.*

Another caregiver explained that his children, who were close in age, also had a delayed reaction to their mother's death several years afterward:

*The issues bubbled to the surface more in the past year than right after. I didn't really anticipate that. My older daughter years later would say, "Remind me of some of the happy times." She was 16 when her mother died; they were butting heads and hadn't resolved their issues.*

*Both girls went back to school, but they kind of wore a tag that put them in a little shell. The older one never let herself even talk much about it. She had some friends who didn't even know how sick her mom had been.*

*We're very close. I speak with the kids every day. They both carry around a great fear of me dying. It's mostly a subtext, but it has been talked about. They have fear of losing a parent again.*

For **Doug's mother**, the challenge became how to help her other son (two years younger) after Doug died:

*Brandon had been struggling for several years after Doug's death. Friends' families would take him on summer vacations with them while Doug was sick, trying to help him have some normalcy.*

*Brandon wanted normalcy for himself, but he went to the high school where Doug had been king. Teachers and everyone there knew Doug. He was in Doug's realm but wanted to hide so he could be Brandon. He changed his friends; those who had been his best buddies were left behind. They were still nice kids that he chose, but he got more into marijuana, etc. We discovered it from his behaviors.*

*Conversation was really important at that time. Brandon was worried about us. He could hear us crying at night and didn't want to worry us, so he tried to power through. The magic of conversation was knowing what times of day would work best for him. He tended not to talk at meals, but late at night or in the car were the more receptive times for him. It turns out that Brandon worried that he'd get cancer when he got to be 14.*

Brandon now goes to a local state university. He lives at home and has developed a nice relationship with his parents, who are getting used to him as an adult. Doug's brother is healthy and getting happier.

**Joe's wife**, who is a nurse in the hospital where he died, found that handling Joe's death was especially hard for her younger son, who was still in high school when his father died:

> The boys always knew Joe as having one illness after another, but he always got better. A few weeks before he died, Joe had been in the hospital with pneumonia and on bypass. Our younger son Matthew absolutely refused to come to the hospital or to talk about it. He was a senior in high school. He was the heartbreak kid right there. Joe was his best friend in the world.
>
> Shortly before he died, Joe said, "I don't think I can keep doing this, but I don't want my boys to think I'm a quitter." I told Matthew he had to go see his dad because I thought Daddy was going to die.
>
> Here he was, a six-foot, 17-year-old kid, and he just collapsed in his daddy's arms. Joe talked to Matthew about sports, which they both loved. He said, "I expect that when you have kids, you'll go out there and coach them, just like I coached you. Do what you want to do, and be what you want to be." Joe died about 36 hours later. I firmly believe that Joe waited until they had had that conversation to die.
>
> Matthew hasn't moved on very well. I've told him that he and his daddy had more good times together in a few years than some people do in a lifetime, and he knows that. Matthew is still at a point of not wanting to get that close again to anyone and get hurt again. A piece of that boy's soul left that day.
>
> When I look back, I think I didn't realize how alone Matthew was throughout Joe's final illness, and I feel bad about that. He had friends and they spent time together, but I learned later that he was afraid to stay in the house alone by himself when I was with his daddy in the hospital. It just breaks my heart, and there's nothing I can do about it.

Like Doug's mother and several of the other caregivers, Joe's wife learned the hard way that it's not just the primary caregiver who struggles with feelings of impending loss as the patient is dying. One of the important jobs of the caregiver is to give those family members who will remain after the patient dies sufficient love, attention, and support at just the time your energy and stamina are taxed to their limits.

Losing a parent is a unique and difficult experience after you've been to college and left home, in part because there aren't a lot of support resources for that age group. **Nora's daughter** explained that:

> *My mother had only two months between diagnosis and passing. She was diagnosed at age 53. I was at UCLA and we had grown up in the Bay area, so I was flying back and forth every weekend. My sister lived in the city. My father was alive and was the real caregiver. I had only had one friend who had lost a parent at that point. You're still establishing who you are in your life, and you don't really know how to deal with all the emotions. It was still in my senior year of college. I hadn't graduated, hadn't gotten married, hadn't had kids—all of these things that you see yourself approaching in your 20s and 30s. For me personally, my relationship had been evolving with my mom and I found that we grew a lot closer as we got older.*
>
> *Personally I struggled to get back to how I felt before, but it never comes back. Then there's a point where you realize you don't want to go back to feeling like it was. For anyone who's young enough to understand what's going on but not old enough to have the emotional skill set to navigate it, losing a parent is heart-wrenching. There aren't any resources for youth in mourning.*

**Claire's daughter** had a similar experience:

> *When you're a teenage girl, you're always bickering with your mother. Then you're away at college for four years. At that point, my mother became my friend. For those couple of years when she was well, we did things together as adults. She had had a difficult life. She was happy and finally starting to enjoy life, and she no longer had a young child to worry about. I never got to spend enough time with her as my friend.*

*It's probably the most difficult thing I'll ever go through in my life. Nothing else could be that bad. I still have days when I feel sorry for myself because she's not around, and I'll be sad that she'll never get to see what I've done.*

For teenagers and young adults who lose a parent before or in the midst of forming adult relationships with them, there remains a void, a hole that feels like the absence of what they had hoped they would have and the lack of a nurturing adult presence in their lives.

For younger children, losing a parent may pose the challenge of never knowing what they missed. This was surely the case for Laurie's daughters, who were eight and five years old when she died. Their story, which follows, is not just about them, but also about a remarkable caregiver who has enriched their lives. It is a testimony to the extraordinary choices some caregivers will make when they decide to serve beyond the call of duty.

Laurie, who was suffering from lymphoma, met Sarah (a nanny and melanoma survivor) while they were sitting by a swimming pool with the children. Laurie had been first diagnosed while pregnant and delivered her second daughter seven weeks early in order to begin chemotherapy. She was separated from her husband now and had no support system except her mother, who lived nearby. Sarah and Laurie became good friends but lost touch after the summer ended.

Two years later and only three months after Laurie had died, her mother was interviewing candidates for a nanny to Laurie's children. During her introductory conversation with Sarah, **Laurie's mother** suddenly threw her hands in the air:

*Oh my God! You're her! Laurie used to tell us about this amazing nanny who was a cancer survivor who was taking care of another family and did all these great things with the kids. My God, here you are! She used to talk with us about you all the time.*

Through her tears, the grandmother then explained that she was really looking for a surrogate mother for the children, Ellie and Amy, now ages eight and five. Because they had been visiting their father when Laurie died and had never even known she had cancer, their caregiving needs would become complicated as they grew up. Believing that there must be "a master plan," **Sarah** took on this demanding role:

> *The girls remembered me from two years before when I had been at the pool with their mother. So I was immediately at school, in the classrooms, doing all the projects. I had to hit the ground running because you can't be the only kid in class whose mom doesn't show up.*

> *Right away I knew that this wasn't just a job. When you're a nanny in this kind of situation, you can't walk off the clock and shut your brain off at six at night and not think about them until the next morning. I worried more about the emotional well-being of those kids than with my past nanny jobs. I just basically acted like a mom. I even talked with the teachers at Christmastime, asking if the class could make gift projects "for your parent" instead of specifically "for Mom."*

> *Most fulfilling has been watching them coming into their own. At a young age, Ellie probably had a lot of responsibility for her little sister Amy while her mother was sick, even though she didn't know it was cancer. For the first year I was with them, the younger one couldn't do anything if her older sister wasn't there.*

> *Now that Ellie isn't solely responsible for Amy, she's come out of her shell and is turning into a bright young woman who is light years away from the quiet little thing I met that day in October five years ago. I had to train Ellie that her job was to be an eight-year-old and go to school and have her own life.*

> *Amy is still afraid of thunderstorms. We made up stories that Mommy is an angel, and when there's thunder, that's when the angels are bowling and Mommy gets a strike. That's how we get through the thunderstorms even today, almost five years later.*

*I do it because those girls need somebody who's there. They didn't see her go through treatment, but they got the worst of it. I'll care about them for the rest of my life, even when I'm no longer their nanny.*

*What I've learned is that being a caregiver takes a lot out of you. I can't stay forever because I can't put my life on hold for too much longer. They'll always be a part of me, but they'll be OK because they're grounded and know where they are and are becoming a little more confident in who they are. At age 13, Ellie now knows about the cancer; she created a Relay For Life team this year to raise money for the American Cancer Society and blew the doors off with her success!*

In a personal conversation several months after her original interview for this book, Sarah shared that Ellie had told her, *I know you're not my mom, but you do everything my mom would have done. You're a really good surrogate mom.* As she helps Laurie's daughters grow up, Sarah has filled an indescribable void in these children's lives and at the same time is being fulfilled in ways she wouldn't have by any ordinary job.

## Resources for Caregivers Concerned About Children

Most resources for caregivers on the topic of engaging the children recommend the approach that many of the interviewees shared—telling the truth but moderating how much truth you tell based on the age of the children, and recognizing that each child will handle that information differently. There are five good resources that can get you started:

- ❧ The American Cancer Society provides suggestions about how to involve and inform children about a cancer diagnosis in the family. Information is also available about how to tell a child that he or she has cancer. Useful links with downloadable information can be found at *www.cancer.org/Treatment* for dealing with these topics.

꿋 The National Cancer Institute (NCI) has a number of publications dealing with how to talk with children about cancer. These can be accessed at *www.cancer.gov/cancertopics/types/childhoodcancers*. These publications also differentiate messages by age group of the children and by severity of the cancer situation.

꿋 Camp Sunshine *(www.campsunshine.org)* is located in Casco, Maine, on the shores of Sebago Lake. As mentioned, this program is free to children with life-threatening illnesses and their immediate families through all stages of their illness. In addition, 24-hour medical and counseling support is available, as are bereavement groups for families who have lost a child to illness. Many other such camps exist nationwide.

꿋 Magical Moon Foundation (MMF) is focused specifically on supporting children and families faced with cancer. Serving children nationwide, MMF focuses on empowering them to find the warrior within. Rather than kids fighting cancer, they become brave young Knights turning their struggles into motivation. Each Knight pursues a project to help build a healthy Earth Kingdom where children won't get cancer. For information, go to *www.magicalmoon.org*.

꿋 A short book, ***Things I Wish I'd Known: Cancer and Kids***, by this author is available at *www.Amazon.com* and *www.thingsiwishidknown.com* and offers a range of child-related resources.

**Doug's mother** offered an inspirational comment to help others through the experience of coaching children through cancer, whether as the patient, a sibling, or a friend:

*Kids are a remarkable breed. It's amazing what they're faced with and can power through, supported by their innocence.*

If you acknowledge this resilience, are honest, and provide unending support, they will get through the cancer experience with grace and surprisingly resilient coping behaviors.

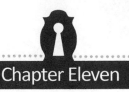

# Chapter Eleven

# Managing Your Emotions and Health

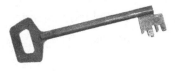

Once a patient has been diagnosed and starts treatment, the plan developed by his medical team offers him certain routines, activities, and milestones. These give him a virtual road map for his experience. They may even give him some sense of what's coming when, and why, to manage his expectations.

In contrast, your life as a caregiver may start to feel quite unpredictable. You're working hard to make sure your patient takes all medications on time, goes to appointments, and remains in good spirits. You're also making sure side effects are managed and communicated to physicians and that the demands of the patient's and your family's day-to-day lives are satisfied. The problem is that there's no real plan to guide you in your role. One day may be quite different from the next.

This chapter deals with the wide range of emotional and physical reactions you're likely to experience and what you might want to do to stay mentally and physically healthy so you can be strong when the going gets tough:

**Sustaining Your Own Emotional and Physical Health**

**Coping Mechanisms for Caregivers**

**Bringing a Patient into Your Home:
Managing the Mixed Blessings**

## Sustaining Your Own Emotional and Physical Health

The unpredictability and volatility of your day-to-day life as a caregiver may take a toll if you're not anticipating its arrival. In response to unexpected patient reactions to a medication, a bad fever, or another potential setback, you're likely to have uncontrollable adrenaline surges. As your hormones kick in to help you rise to the challenge of the new perceived emergency, your heart will start pumping, anxiety will increase, and you may find that you just can't calm down. The closer you are in relationship and/or proximity to the patient, the more reactive you're likely to become, and the less in control you may feel.

Then, once the "high" of the fast response wears off, you may find yourself feeling exhausted, lethargic, or depressed—until the next challenge. Before long, you may even find yourself multi-tasking to the point of losing things, making mistakes in activities you know well, driving too fast, or even falling asleep in a doctor's waiting room. Such an emotional and hormonal roller coaster can become debilitating over time.

As the pace and unpredictability increase, it will be too easy to overlook your own support needs. If you're anything like many of the interviewees, you may find yourself simply putting one foot in front of the other, trying to keep a steady course and working hard not to show your own emotional reactions for fear of adding to your patient's level of anxiety.

Research has shown that cancer caregivers faced with such challenges are more likely to neglect their own health than the rest of the population. They develop poor eating habits, demonstrate higher fatigue levels, have worse exercise and sleep habits, and display more symptoms of depression than before they began the journey. More than one in 10 caregivers reported that caregiving caused their physical health to deteriorate.[32] One academic study estimated that the stress of caregiving can take as many as 10 years off a family caregiver's life.[33]

For these reasons, you need to pay attention to your own well-being and make sure you don't run yourself ragged. After all, your patient and family depend on you, and you can't remain strong and alert in the face of the many demands of the cancer journey if you don't take care of yourself. For example, it took a mini-lecture from his son's surgeon to convince **Michael S's father** that he needed rest after his son's lengthy surgery:

> *I had taken care of everything in the family for years. The night after the surgery, when I'd had no sleep for 26 hours and the surgery had taken 14 hours, I was leaning on a radiator outside our son's room. The surgeon came by at 4 a.m., and he looked really good.*
>
> *I asked him how he looked so good after a 14-hour surgery, and he said he'd taken a shower. He added, "I feel a lot better. Now I'm going home to sleep. Your son will be unconscious for 12 hours. Nurses here are the best. If you don't take care of yourself, they will have to take care of you. You'll be no good to your son if you collapse physically, mentally, or emotionally. You won't see it coming.*

While many caregivers believe that it's OK for their patients to feel sad, afraid, or anxious, they don't give themselves permission to do so because they think they're supposed to be strong for their patient. Yet there is no emotional reaction that is inappropriate or out of line. Caregivers have experienced them all but have remained effective. What's important is identifying the impact your emotions are having on your own health and well-being and on your ability to care for your patient.

---

32  "How do Family Caregivers Fare? A Closer Look at their Experiences," Center on Aging Society, 2005, quoted at *www.thefamilycaregiver.org*.

33  Elissa S. Epel, Department of Psychiatry, University of California S.F., *et. al.*, from the Proceedings of the National Academy of Sciences, December 7, 2004, Vol. 101, No. 49, quoted at *www.thefamilycaregiver.org*.

Your reactions are what they are. Allow friends and other support resources to listen but not to judge you or your feelings. It's not a weakness to admit that your own emotional or physical symptoms are interfering with your functioning as an effective caregiver; it *is* a weakness to refuse to recognize your own limits.

The most important principle that cancer caregivers shared is that you know yourself better than anyone else, so you need to identity and think about:

- ∽ What emotions you are experiencing: fear, anger, guilt, sadness, confusion, anxiety, being overwhelmed, and so on.

- ∽ What physical reactions you are feeling: racing heartbeat, exhaustion, sleep deprivation, sagging energy level, and so on.

- ∽ Whether professional, psychological, or medical help could ease those symptoms so you can be a more effective caregiver.

- ∽ Whether airing your feelings will help or hurt you.

A fairly common characteristic of cancer caregivers is that they feel strong emotions but bottle them up. Some couples find the cancer experience so emotionally threatening that their coping behavior is "radio silence."

A year after he completed cancer treatment, **Brad and his wife** were barely speaking. A local doctor, he had decided on his own not to tell even their friends about their cancer ordeal, inadvertently isolating his wife. As a result, they each withdrew and never discussed their respective feelings during and after his treatment.

One day, with the help of an oncology social worker, she overcame her tears and talked through her feelings. When she returned home that evening, Brad could tell from her body language that something had changed. His asking "How did it go?" (for the first time) reopened dialogue and allowed them to share their stifled emotional reactions to his illness, saving their marriage.

While understandable, such stoicism isn't always the best way to proceed, although there are times when it can prove helpful.

As a serial caregiver, **Chuck and Laura's brother** found that caring for one sibling who had died and then having to care for another who was dying, in rapid succession, made it nearly impossible for him to vent his feelings in ways that would relieve the stress:

> *My caregiving energies that I had focused on my brother transferred to his wife, his daughter, and our parents. I'd say to them, "I'm here. You've been through a lot more than I." I'm a control guy, and I was losing a second sibling. I had little time or energy to get rid of the anger.*
>
> *I ended up going on, because every time I wanted to feel sorry for myself, I'd look at my mother and father, each in a different chapter in the book of grief. A parent losing a child isn't just in a different book—the parent is in a differentli-brary. I said to myself that I didn't have the right to complain about my own grief.*

Even though he had been a rock in caring for his brother, he subsequently learned the hard way that he needed to care for himself while caring for his next patient:

> *Each cancer patient gets concerned that his disease is killing you. My sister was worried about me, as was my mom. I made myself get some sleep just to ease their worry. If you're a serious caregiver rather than a flash in the pan, you have to learn how to care for yourself and keep your battery charged because you'll be doing lots of things you normally don't do.*

**Jack's daughter**, whose siblings were happy for her to fill the primary caregiver's role, both for her father who suffered from prostate cancer and for her suicidal mother, didn't realize at the time how much support she really needed:

> *I was surprised that I often slept like a rock. I could not have sustained my stamina without it. I shuttled our mom back and forth to the hospital, dropped the kids off at school, took*

*care of Mom, visited my father, and occasionally swapped with my siblings. I was the primary caregiver, and I was going on autopilot.*

When asked whether her two sisters ever inquired how she was doing in the midst of such a chaotic series of events, she started to cry. Wiping her tears, she shook her head and replied:

*I was in survival and self-preservation mode. My siblings never asked how I was doing, and I never asked for help. I never dealt with the emotional part of it, so it still comes out at unexpected times.*

For **Tiffany's husband,** the routine of daily life and caring for their young son kept him from having to face his fears and emotions:

*It was better not to be alone in my thoughts. It was easier that way. I could worry about our one-year-old son's needs and take my mind off of my own. There was some comfort in the routines that I had to go through with him and the fact that they didn't allow me to have time on my own. I couldn't let myself feel tired.*

But **Tiffany** had a different point of view, wishing that her caregiver husband could have shown more emotion during her cancer battle:

*My husband ended up with an ulcer while caring for me; he didn't cry except when with his own family. It would have helped me if he'd cried in my presence just once. It would have felt like we were really together in the ordeal.*

**Bobbi**, a 20-year breast cancer survivor, had a similar reaction:

*Caregivers haven't experienced physical pain and can't make it go away, so they have to be inventive. They feel the need to be strong, but sometimes that strength is protective armor. It would have helped my healing process for my husband to have revealed his real feelings with me every so often. I know he did it with the kids, but it would have helped me to understand how the experience had affected him.*

Some other caregivers let their emotions out but were careful to choose their time and place. For **Paul's wife**, it was important to acknowledge that they were there:

> Recognize that your fear and emotional reactions are OK. They're normal. The period of being lonely and bored was short, but the anxiety was big. It was the unknown future and wondering if I would become a widow. It was hard to deal with, but it never got in the way of my functioning until the very end. I had held it together until we were nearing the end of treatments, when I had time to just fall apart.
>
> No one had talked with me about what it would feel like to be the caregiver, but my therapist validated that my feelings weren't unusual.

Even negative feelings are to be expected, acknowledged, and respected. One caregiver nearly got into a bar fight one evening before he recognized his level of stress. Another felt the pain of her husband's potentially terminal diagnosis so strongly that she actually considered running away:

> At one point, I said to my husband that I'm not helping at all and maybe I should just leave. I think it's because I was so scared of loss and the idea of leaving was the way to avoid it.

Then she realized that she was just feeling overwhelmed. It's hard to flee from cancer when you're looking after someone you care about, although fantasies of escape from the burden are common.

Several caregivers experienced guilt but felt bad about expressing it. Sharon's daughter survived leukemia. A year later, she was diagnosed with metastatic breast cancer. **Sharon's sister** described her own reaction:

> No matter how much you do, you'll feel guilty for being healthy, for not doing more, for not having chemo. Guilty that you can't fix it. Guilty for having healthy children. Worried about what's going to happen to me. If someone had told me that in the beginning, it would have made me feel a little better. You can't not be those things, so acknowledge it and let it go as much as possible.

**Tommy's sister** is still upset about not having had the chance to say good-bye more than 13 years ago when her brother died suddenly of a stroke after surgery for brain cancer. She was crying when she explained:

> I feel guilt. The night before he died, I was watching TV—Garth Brooks, who was Tommy's favorite. I wondered if he was watching it. It was 9:30 and I didn't want to bother him. I wish I'd called. I don't know if he knew how much I loved him.
>
> The next morning I saw one of my sisters and then went to work. I was one of the last to arrive after he died, and I didn't learn for 13 years that when I saw her earlier in the day, my sister had known that he was dying but hadn't told me. I remember the days of the funeral, his death, his wake like they were yesterday.

**Joe's wife**, a nurse, felt guilty she hadn't been able to save her husband, even though he had been sick with one problem or another for all of their 30 years of married life. An important insight from a psychiatrist helped her put those feelings into perspective:

> As a nurse or physician, you feel guilty because you're supposed to be able to fix it. You can't be everything to everybody, and you feel so guilty, or you think, "Man, I've missed this" or "I should have been there for that" or "I didn't get to do something," but they're only feelings. As long as you're doing the right thing, don't beat yourself up.

**Judy O's husband** spent days at the hospital after his wife caught a staph infection there following her breast cancer surgery. Unbeknownst to him, the combination of worry and long hours took its toll:

> After 35 days in the hospital, when I'd been there from nine in the morning until nine at night, I thought I was doing pretty well. I was driving home on the Expressway one night at 9 p.m. All of a sudden I started to weep. I pulled over into the breakdown lane. A state trooper stopped behind me five minutes later and looked in. When he asked what was wrong,

> *I told him my story, and he said, "Take your time." He direct-*
> *ed traffic around me. When I was ready to leave, I got out of*
> *the car and I told him I never thought I'd have my breakdown*
> *in the breakdown lane. That's Irish humor for you.*

The state trooper followed him the remaining 20 miles home to make sure he got there in one piece. That incident helped Judy's husband realize how he had neglected himself.

Numerous caregivers recognized that an intense caregiving experience brings with it both positive and negative surprises. Their common suggestion was not to let either highs or lows take you along. **Jacqueline's husband** said:

> *I stayed even-keeled throughout the caregiving. I never let*
> *the highs get too high or the lows get too low. We celebrated*
> *good news and mitigated the bad news.*

Between the lines, caregivers also suggested that you avoid jumping to conclusions. A piece of good news doesn't mean the patient is out of the woods any more than a setback means he'll die. As **Chuck's brother** said: *It's not an event—it's a process.*

The important lesson from these stories is that family caregiving for a cancer patient can be an intensely trying and emotional experience. You'll be healthier and more resilient during the process if you acknowledge your feelings and figure out how and when to let them out. As **Mindy's husband** said after he'd been coping with his wife's uncertain prognosis for more than 18 months:

> *Accept your emotions for what they are and allow yourself to*
> *have them so you can move on. Be upset that life will change*
> *permanently, and then get over it. Don't squash your emotions.*
>
> *We were pissed off that it happened to us. We despaired that*
> *we couldn't do what we'd planned. Don't let the anger pre-*
> *vent you from doing what needs to be done. Do things, even*
> *if life won't be perfect.*

## Coping Mechanisms for Caregivers

Many caregivers are tempted to throw every ounce of their energy into caregiving. It's normal to feel as though the odds of success increase with every hour that you devote to patient care. The temptation to give up or greatly curtail one's daily routine can be overwhelming, as can the feeling that wanting a few minutes "off duty" is a sign of selfishness. It's difficult for a caregiver to deal with the fact that he has no control over the situation. As **Mike S's wife** explained, *I could never say to Mike, "I'll take the cancer for an hour. You take a break."*

Most of the caregivers who contributed to this book experienced such feelings, but **Jen P's husband** put them in context:

> *You could really let yourself go, but I'd read enough to know I had to take care of myself first. On an airplane, they tell you when the oxygen masks fall down, put the mask on yourself first and your kids second. I had to stay physically fit and give myself a mental break to run or play golf. Otherwise it could drive you kooky.*

### Work and Everyday Activities

For some caregivers, it was work that kept them feeling competent and as if their lives were under control:

> **Ed's wife** *Work was a helpful escape. I can't imagine how intense it would be to stay home as a full-time caregiver.*

> **John D's daughter** *Actually, work became a distraction and an escape. My boss said that you can't be there 24/7, and coming here can give you a break.*

> **Tim N's wife** *I'm a partner in a law firm. Work was soothing and predictable for me. I knew how to do it and that I was good at it. It was very comforting. I couldn't sleep a lot when he was sick. I'd wake up in the middle of the night, at two in the morning, and I'd lie there completely terrified.*

*So I'd get up and start working, and it would make me feel calmer so I could go back to sleep.*

**Jen P's husband** discovered during his wife's treatment that his nighttime fears would melt away when he had to focus on the requirements of day-to-day living:

*There were certainly nights when I'd lie in bed and think about what life would be like if I lose her. All kinds of crazy thoughts would go through my mind, like what will I do with the kids, and how will I raise my daughter without her mother, and it's not fair. Then I'd wake up in the morning and take a shower and life stuff would take over, and I'd forget about the hypothetical stuff. As you get farther away from it, the bad nights get fewer and farther between.*

Some caregivers were more deliberate about engaging in everyday activities that would provide relief from their caregiving burdens. **Tom's wife** emphasized how important it was to maintain interest in other parts of your life:

*Don't quit your book club, or your garden club. Don't quit your own interests. You have to keep going and get away from it and keep thinking about other things. You can't do all cancer all the time. You need to live a life.*

**Lynn's husband** had retired to spend more time with her and to provide her care, but as he did so, she looked out for his mental health:

*One saving grace was that she made me keep my early morning ritual. Every morning I used to jump in the truck, go to the local coffee shop to pick up the dirty joke of the day, drive around the reservoir and see the ducks, and then go home. She insisted that I keep doing that. She knew how important it was to me. I hated driving back into the driveway because the pressure would start up as soon as I walked back in the door.*

*Working could have diverted some of the pressure, but it did help not to have the added stress of the job. I started a new project building a model of an old fishing schooner. I was into it and had to work on small pieces for hours. It required intense concentration and problem-solving but we could both be in the same place (living room). I only realized the value of the project as a diversion later.*

## Hobbies, Exercise, and Mindless Activities

Many caregivers found respite in the form of a wide variety of diversions. For **Jim D's daughter**, who was caring for both parents in their home at a distance from her family, it was walking their dog or going to the supermarket. Others used reading, painting, writing poetry, or even folding laundry (truly a thought-free activity!) to take their minds off the cancer fight.

**Amelia's husband** incorporated his hobby into his caregiving role:

*I'm a photographer. I started photographing Amelia during her illness, but I have the pictures in a drawer and can't bring myself to touch them yet. It was helpful in documenting the experience because so few people understand what it was like. My pictures and my journal capture it so it doesn't bounce around in my head and make me crazy. When it happens, it feels like nobody knows what you're going through.*

*Amelia was receptive to my doing it, but the process created conflicting feelings: on the one hand of capturing something so personal at the expense of my wife, and on the other hand feeling it might be useful to other people.*

**Tracy's husband** is a business executive with a musical bent:

*I'm a musician in my spare time. I play drums. For me, that was my therapy. My band practiced three nights a week, and I looked forward to going to see my friends, sitting down, having a beer, and playing the drums.*

*Cancer wasn't there. I had to focus on the music to make it sound right. A couple of hours on those nights, I'd walk out of there and sleep better. I didn't think about Tracy, school, work, cancer. It all went away. When I put the drumsticks down after practice, I felt better. I could hit the drums as hard as I had to in order to get out the frustrations.*

**Trudy's domestic partner** maintained her long-term hobby despite the volatility of Trudy's condition:

*My sanity comes from volunteering for 13 years with the Northeast Canine Search & Rescue organization. We train our own dogs to track and identify human scent off lead in the woods. I get the dog in the right place and he does the work. I train with the dog two or three times a week and am on call 24/7. My only time away from Trudy is when I'm doing this. A few friends help when I'm on duty. My sanity comes from this, and my relationship with my dog is huge.*

Several caregivers used different forms of exercise as diversions, pursuing sports like karate and golf, which require intense concentration and offer a way to let out both tension and feelings of anger. For **Mindy's husband**, it was competitive biking:

*My bike riding was important. I started doing longer routes, so it became an athletic endeavor. Do your best, but also escape. Sometimes I'd spend three hours not having to care for anyone or worrying about what would happen. Mindy understood that it was for relief.*

Initially neither Mindy's mother nor his own appreciated his need to lose himself in biking, but **Mindy** herself was his greatest cheerleader:

*Our mothers passed judgment on him when he took bike rides or went to a soccer game with the kids. He stopped riding for weeks because of what he felt was the way they looked at him. "Everyone tells me to take time for myself, but no one lets me do it," he said.*

*Sometimes he'd lie and say he had to grade papers. He felt as if he was doing something seemingly selfish, but the word "selfish" isn't a bad thing. He had self-knowledge. I had things being done to me, but he had to structure his caregiving experience.*

*When he'd come back from bike riding, he'd look like his old self and sleep better. The thing about biking is that he could do it on his own and not need a partner or a team. Neighborhood bikers helped him learn where to ride, how to repair a bike, and so on. He didn't have to talk about himself or my situation.*

*At one point he did a century ride—100 miles in six hours. His mom took the kids and saw him at the course. She was much more supportive after seeing how positive it made him feel.*

There is no doubt that taking care of yourself is central to cancer caregiving. Just as important is articulating that need openly so others on the caregiving team understand and can be supportive.

### Talking With Others

A number of caregivers found that their greatest stress relief came from talking to others who were going through a similar situation:

**Mike S's wife** *I often took a walk with a friend whose husband had ALS. Our experiences were remarkably parallel both practically and emotionally.*

**Doug's mother** *I took time-outs to hike or go somewhere. It would have helped me if I'd taken time for my own self-reflection, but I didn't. It also helped to have a neutral voice, a 1-800 voice, to answer questions, like the American Cancer Society's national call information center.*

**David's sister** *People at Hope Lodge would ask, "How are you?" I took time to express what was going on and let HL folks help. When you open yourself up to others and are there for them, you become stronger. I had wonderful experiences in supporting other patients in treatment and their caregivers.*

*You're just more balanced, instead of being overtired and distraught. You're very aware that you're not alone.*

Stress relief for some came from talking to a counselor, mental health professional, or support group. For example, while **John's daughter** was primary caregiver for her father, who was suffering from mesothelioma, she sought help and support for other battles she had to fight at the same time:

*I saw a counselor regularly. It helped me deal with my anger at the insurance company, which was giving us problems with Dad's insurance. The counselor was able to allow me to let it out by yelling and crying, so I could keep it under control in other settings. The counselor said, "The lifeguard has to stay physically and mentally fit or he can't save a life."*

**Ned's wife** realized in hindsight that a social worker would have been helpful for herself in order to be able to give her husband what he needed:

*In many ways, the caregiver needs a social worker as much as the patient. Ned and I went together a few times. Ned finally said to me that it was easier for him not to talk about it. While it made it much more difficult for me, I began to realize that was how it needed to be for him. I went a few times alone but I think it might have been beneficial to go alone regularly to process what was going on and to have a reality check when I began to feel like I was going crazy or overwhelmed.*

With only a few exceptions, most caregivers found that it mattered less what form of stress reliever they chose and more that it reminded them of life B.C. (before cancer), so they could endure the caregiving marathon.

## Bringing a Patient into Your Home: Managing the Mixed Blessings

When you consider bringing a cancer patient into your own home for the later stages of life, you need to prepare for one of the most dramatic combinations of positive and negative emotions that arise almost simultaneously. **Artie's daughter-in-law** described an intense example of bringing her father-in-law into her home as he was dying from mesothelioma. This *"extreme challenge"* tested everything she holds dear, but she wouldn't have traded it for any alternative that was available. Her description was articulate, vivid, and caring, and it should be useful for managing your expectations if you are considering such a caregiving situation:

> *It was an extreme challenge in more ways than one to have my husband's father living in the house during his treatment. Initially Artie had a really good three or four months when he was fine. He couldn't drive, but he still did what he wanted to do.*
>
> *Then he got on oxygen, which meant that he had to have the tank with him, so he couldn't just run out and go. We had a big machine for use in the house that had a long cord so he could get around. We gave him our son's room and our son (who was eight) moved downstairs so Artie could be on one floor once we got him in the house.*
>
> *Artie was a stubborn little Italian dad. He didn't want to be a burden and asked to be put in a "hospice home," but my husband Charlie wouldn't hear of that.*
>
> *Day-to-day, the hardest thing for me was when he couldn't get on and off the toilet. It was just him and me. What am I going to do? So I said, "Artie, I don't mind if you don't mind." He said, "I feel so bad for you." He was embarrassed. It got to the point where I had to literally pick him up from the toilet and help him get his pants back on. I said, "I'm not going to look." Charlie would give him a sponge bath or a shower, and we had a seat for him in the shower.*
>
> *I remember one time he was in the hospital bed. We had regular twin sheets, but they don't fit the mattress, so I ran over to Wal-Mart as quickly as I could. By the time I got back, he was in tears because he had to go to the bathroom so badly and he had thought he was going to mess his pants. He had*

*prayed to the Lord the whole time I was gone and then asked could I please help him get into the bathroom. It was things like that [issues of human dignity] that were really hard.*

*The stress on the nuclear family, the five of us, was nothing like I've ever experienced. Every little dynamic of your house changes. Not just the physical things like the grocery bills going way up, and cooking and doing laundry for an extra person, but your whole life, like with the kids. I have a five-year-old who wants her dinner, but I have a 77-year-old man who needs my help. You're always pulled in different directions.*

*You're so bone tired at the end of the day that if you're able to sleep, you'll sleep like a rock and are afraid you won't hear if he needs help. So we set up a baby monitor, and that worked wonderfully. He could call down and tell us what he needed —medicine, or pills, or to have his drains emptied.*

*Charlie's number one was his dad. He was so emotional that I honestly wondered if we'd still be married after all of this. He's a screamer, so he'd yell and scream over something stupid that had nothing to do with anything. I just told the kids that, "Mommy and Daddy aren't ourselves right now. We're very stressed and very sad, and you're great helpers."*

*I met with the pediatrician ahead of time and explained what we were doing and asked what he recommended. He said you're teaching the children a wonderful thing, what family is and what they do for each other. In that aspect, it was good, but honestly I couldn't begin to put into words how stressful it was.*

*Home care is 24/7. There were times when I got almost resentful. My bathroom has a gorgeous vanity in it, and we had to put his oxygen under it, so I couldn't dry my hair, or do my makeup. The first day I realized that, I started to cry. It felt like I didn't even get one little piece of my house. It was something stupid like drying my hair, but I had a lump in my throat and was stomping my feet and moving my stuff. We had to find a different place for everything, to the point where the dog food was kept in that bathroom. I think that people who haven't been through it have no idea how that feels.*

*Of all the caregiving I've done, this was the most stressful. I learned as I went, plus it was in my home. At the end, Artie just kept saying, "Send me to the hospice house. What if I die?" and I said, "We'll be right here holding your hand. We want you here with us."*

Every caregiver's home care experience is stressful in different ways:

- For **Annie's husband**, home care meant setting up hospital-like arrangements so he could empty drains, give injections, change surgical dressings, and clean surgical wounds that just wouldn't heal.

- For **Jenn S's husband**, it meant keeping a bucket and a bottle of fresh water next to the bed, as well as a spare set of sheets easily accessible in case she was sick during the night. (Fortunately, the bucket has been retired.)

- **Jacqueline's husband** says proudly that, *She was only in the hospital the day she died. I washed her and bathed her and washed her clothes.*

Still others were consumed in child care, or preparing special meals, or just being there. What matters is that every home care situation is its own. For some, it's just a temporary phase of life, and for others it's working through a terminal situation with help from hospice staff.

Caring for a cancer patient at home can be enormously rewarding. Several of the caregivers said it helped them feel like they had done everything possible for their patients in keeping them comfortable and relaxed throughout their cancer experiences. This was true regardless of the patient's outcome.

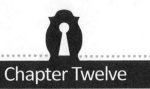

# Chapter Twelve

# Nearing Life's End

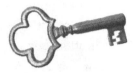

Some patients end up living with cancer and undergo various treatments over time as new treatments become available. The longer they live, the greater their hope. Others, and there are more of them every day, become cancer-free and emerge from their treatment as survivors. Still others decline when their cancers no longer respond to available therapies. Those patients and their caregivers are confronted with planning for symptom relief and a probable death.

Difficult conversations can happen at any point during a caregiving experience. They may come as early as telling family members about the diagnosis or as late as having a significant discussion about funeral arrangements while the patient is still rational. Still, the final stages often bring with them some of the most sensitive and challenging exchanges.

Talking through some of these difficult issues ahead of time can make it easier for both patient and caregiver alike. In that regard, this chapter deals with:

**Advance Directives for Extraordinary Measures**

**Decisions to Stop Treatment and/or to Activate Hospice**

**Difficult Conversations about Death and Dying**

**The Lasting Impact of Unexpected Kindnesses**

**Helping a Patient to Die With Dignity**

There are many resources available to support patients who are being cared for at home:

- 🦐 The National Cancer Institute (*www.cancer.gov*) provides a useful overview of the kinds of medical and logistical resources that may be available in your community. Medical resources may include registered nurses, physical therapists, and social workers, while other services might include medical equipment (hospital bed, oxygen tanks, and so on), licensed home health aides (for help in dressing or bathing patients, preparing meals, and delivery of medication), or providers of complementary therapies like yoga or massage.

- 🦐 The American Cancer Society provides overview information about such home health resources online at *www.cancer.org*.

- 🦐 Medicare also provides a potentially useful website (*www.medicare.gov/HomeHealthCompare*) for sourcing home health and equipment agencies.

- 🦐 The National Association for Home Care and Hospice (*www.nahc.org*) provides consumer information about how to choose an agency, how they work, how they bill, and other useful information that may be helpful in planning for home care arrangements.

## Advance Directives for Extraordinary Measures

Advance directives are decisions made ahead of time and conveyed in legal documents which can be activated in the event that the patient becomes too ill to communicate clearly with the medical team. They provide a sense of security for both patients and caregivers that the patient's wishes will be respected and confusion or mistakes minimized.

Advance directives can be revised as long as the changes are signed and notarized in a legal manner when the patient is conscious and of sound mind. If the patient is unable to get changes made in writing, his direct verbal instructions will generally suffice. Because laws vary from state to state, be sure to check the relevant provisions that apply, perhaps with the help of a hospital's social worker, a health care navigator, or your own attorney.

As caregiver, it is important to keep copies of any advance directives. Upon any hospital admission, make sure that they are in the patient's file or provide a copy so that the medical staff knows the patient's preferences regarding treatment.

There are three main kinds of directives:

- 🙟 Living Will
- 🙟 Durable Power of Attorney (POA) for health care
- 🙟 Do Not Resuscitate (DNR) order

A useful resource that explains the advantages and disadvantages of each of these documents and how to get them drafted is *www.caregiver.org*, the website of the Family Caregiver Alliance. A good resource for obtaining forms for your state is *www.compassionindying.org*.

## Living Will

Health care institutions are in the business of keeping patients alive for as long as possible. As a result, the medical team will use all available means necessary to prolong life—from cardiopulmonary resuscitation (mechanical pressure on the chest to restore heart rhythm), to defibrillators which shock the heart back into beating, to feeding tubes, repeated blood transfusions, respirators, dialysis, and other kinds of life-supporting machines.

Some patients don't want their lives to be extended, especially if it means being hooked up to machines and may result in diminished or inferior quality of life. A living will is a legal document that instructs caregivers and medical service providers what actions to take—or not take—to prolong a patient's life at a time when the patient becomes incapable of making necessary decisions for himself.

Because discussions about advance directives tend to feel awkward during a critical illness, the ideal time to have them is before a cancer diagnosis.

Barring that, the best alternative is to conduct conversations early on about whether to take extraordinary measures to save the patient's life.

**Mike S's wife** initiated those talks at a time that would generate less emotional turmoil for the family:

> I had conversations with Mike's oncologist using euphemisms about "reasonable vs. heroic measures." To the degree possible, if death is likely, caregivers should think through how to handle things so you and your family are all on the same page. Make sure you all agree on the interpretation of what the patient actually wants for the end of life.
>
> A health care proxy is very important. Mike wanted to have options, but he knew when enough was enough. It can be shattering if you don't talk about it ahead of time. The conversations are painful because you have to acknowledge the inevitable, but my advice is to do it sooner, rather than later.

**George's daughter** also felt that advance directives should have been considered early on in his illness. The fact that they were not in place made having the conversation late in his illness awkward, if not impossible:

> We didn't talk about—and I wish we had—what arrangements to make when it happens. By the time we discovered that his cancer had metastasized, he didn't want to talk about dying. We could have talked before, but not when death was imminent.
>
> There comes a point where you have to make decisions for care, comfort, and convenience for everybody that may not be consistent with the patient's wants. It's the best you can do. There's no perfect way to deal with the situation. You just have to do your best. You get as much data as possible, but ultimately you have to make the decision.

Ideally, advance directives are legal planning tools that all of us should have, preferably formulated when we're healthy. They're even more important when someone is embarking on an uncertain and often unpredictable experience like the cancer journey. The documents can sit in a file folder so long as you don't need them, but you'll be grateful that you have them when the time comes.

**Durable Power of Attorney for Health Care**

With a durable power of attorney (often known as a POA or durable power) for health care, the patient designates someone else to make decisions on his behalf in the event that he is unable to make them for himself. That individual is known as the patient's health care proxy or stand-in. A durable POA may be more versatile than a simple living will because it empowers someone chosen by the patient to make needed decisions when conditions are changing rapidly. That person is usually the caregiver, but it may also be someone else, such as another member of the family.

It should be noted that a durable POA for health care doesn't authorize the proxy to handle the patient's financial affairs. If the patient chooses to include making financial decisions, that directive can be incorporated or created as a separate document.

In the end, a patient's preferences may not cover every situation that will arise. You may be called on to make decisions that run counter to his written instructions. That's what happened to **Trudy's sister**:

> *The hardest part is dealing with the unknown—what's next and what will the future be like. For instance, Trudy had said she wanted no blood transfusions, but when she needed surgery for broken bones, the surgeon said he wouldn't operate if she couldn't have transfusions. By the time we learned she needed a transfusion, she was drugged up and couldn't be consulted, so we just did the transfusion and moved on.*

**Do Not Resuscitate (DNR) Order**

Because standard protocol in any health care facility is to do everything possible to sustain life, including bringing a patient back from the brink of death, a Do Not Resuscitate (DNR) Order is a legal request not to use any restorative measures if the patient's heartbeat or breathing stops and his condition is dire or terminal. Some patients will initiate such an order to reduce potential suffering for themselves and their loved ones and to give them a feeling of control over their dying process.

All three of the legal documents mentioned are best prepared early because the need for them may arise suddenly when there is little time to make the necessary legal arrangements.

Tim S was faced with the unexpected prospect of urgent brain surgery. He and his wife had to do fast contingency planning even before they knew how his diagnosis and treatment would evolve. **Tim's wife** explained that:

> *The night before his surgery, I went into his room. Tim was very clear that if he survived the surgery but wasn't "OK," he didn't want to live. He wanted no extraordinary measures to keep him alive if he were to suffer severe brain damage. The next morning it was a comedy of errors to get the forms completed and witnessed before his surgery.*

Annie also initiated conversation with her husband about not wanting anyone to use heroic measures to keep her alive at the end of her life. **Annie's husband** says that:

> *About a week before she died, she told me that if they ever have to use the paddles on her, "I don't want them to do it anymore. My body has lost the fight. I just want them to leave me alone. Just tell them not to try to bring me back. Don't give me anything anymore. I don't want it."*

It's essential that caregivers make sure that a DNR is attached to the patient's medical records at all times in order to guarantee compliance. Skilled nursing or rehabilitation hospital facilities may incorporate advance directives into their files, but they don't always send them along with the patient in an ambulance if there is an emergency hospitalization. Sometimes health care professionals may also overlook a DNR or other advance directive that is in the file, so the caregiver's reminders are critical.

## Decisions to Stop Treatment and/or to Activate Hospice

In terminal situations, the physician, patient, or caregiver may ask to skip curative treatments while continuing to relieve pain or suffering, and the option may arise to move the patient into a hospice setting. Hospice care is focused on improving the quality of life for patients who are dying and to relieve stress for their family caregivers.[34] It is intended to make them as comfortable as possible for a period of time that can be as short as a few days or as long as six months. Depending on the patient's condition and needs, such services may be provided at home or in small hospice facilities, skilled nursing facilities (known as SNFs), or a hospital.

Every hospice operates differently. You're likely to be dealing with a number of nurses, so ensure that there is a single case manager and that the nurses are taking preventive measures to avoid bed sores and to provide bowel care for patients who are immobilized. These actions are critical to quality of life for both the patient and the family.

For **Susan's daughters**, the decision to stop treatment for her brain tumor came when they realized that her quality of life had deteriorated to the point that further efforts might give her a few more weeks or months, but could be difficult for her to tolerate:

> We had an appointment with the neuro-oncologist to discuss what could be the next steps. At this point Mom was in a wheelchair. We were lifting her and moving her for everything. Her mind wasn't what it had been, and she was moving in and out of reality. She was quiet but answered the doctor's questions. If she had a question, it took so long for her to articulate it that she'd forget what question she wanted to ask.
>
> The family had a conversation about quality of life. Given available chemo treatments and statistics and her situation, they said there was a 10% chance of her staying where she was and not deteriorating any further. Continuing with treatment

---

34  See *www.mayoclinic.com* or *www.nlm.nih.gov* and search "hospice."

*would be torture. She had moments of realization of what was happening, and when she did, she would be sobbing.*

*Dad wanted to try everything, but to keep her in the current state seemed cruel. We talked to Dad and said, "Mom has done her job. She raised us and we're adults. We had*

*35 and 36 years with her. She did her job. Our job now is to get her through her journey as humanely and lovingly as we can to make it OK." Our decision was not to do the chemo. We had to talk him into that, but it was the right thing to do for her.*

John's family had hope that a lung transplant would sustain his life. His daughter even offered one of her own lungs, but the odds of rejection were too high because his blood was too healthy. The option of putting him on formal chemotherapy to lower the risk of rejection might have given him another five to eight years to live, but according to **John's daughter**:

*He decided not to proceed with treatment. He wouldn't agree to taking my lung because he said I still had my whole life to live. Even if he did the transplant, it would be an ordeal— he would have had to spend a lot of time in isolation in the hospital more than two hours away from home. Instead, he wanted the quality of life that he had already. We understood his decision. His philosophy was that every day is a different day, and you live it to the fullest. "This is just a bump in the road," he'd say, "but tomorrow will be a different day." He had a positive attitude for all of it.*

Going to a hospice for the last days, weeks, or months of a patient's life or having hospice professionals come to the patient's home to help in his care can be a surprisingly positive experience. Although it comes at a very difficult time, having professional caregivers present during the last stage of life can provide much needed support for both patient and family.

For **Frank B's son**, the decision to call hospice came sooner than he or his family expected, when a young female oncologist advised him to do so. Even though he wasn't ready to accept his father's terminal situation, he found the hospice services to be helpful in managing the family's expectations about the dying process:

> I felt so alone. It felt like I was the only one experiencing this kind of thing. Hospice was the only avenue that let me express my feelings and not have to talk. It was all happening too fast to know what to ask. It was like rope running through my hands.

> When something like this happens, you think of your own mortality really fast. Hospice gave us "The Little Blue Book" and suggested we read it. You don't want to read it, but when things start to change, you go to it. It was eerie how specific it was in terms of physical changes to expect. One of my sisters was changing his sheets, and she noticed that his legs were changing color. It was a rallying point when he seemed lucid and normal. At times like that, "The Little Blue Book" kept us from getting false hopes.

Although hospice services help relieve stress and manage the patient's dying process, caregivers still spend considerable time and energy alongside hospice workers. The Rosalynn Carter Institute for Caregiving attests that "family caregivers of terminally ill cancer patients report providing an average of 115 hours of care each week and report depressive symptoms and health problems far in excess of age-matched controls."[35] Grief counseling is often available through Hospice after the patient's death.

**Amelia's husband** says that he and their daughters were her primary caregivers but that hospice resources gave them many kinds of support and guidance:

> During hospice, we took turns around the clock. The girls would take days off and alternate until the last two weeks, when we all stopped working. The hospice nurse visited three times a week for an hour each time.

> We were the boat and hospice staff was the rudder. They showed us how to administer medications and told us what to watch for. We were treating her to keep her comfortable,

---

35 *www.rosalynncarter.org.*

*and they taught us how to do that. At the end, we had a home health aide who was found through hospice. They prepared us for the dying process and even gave spiritual support. Afterwards we could have had ongoing support if we'd chosen to take it. It wasn't a piece of cake; we cry and we laugh, but we keep going.*

There are several useful resources for learning more about hospice care in your local area:

∽ The National Cancer Institute provides an overview of hospice at *www.nlm.nih.gov.*

∽ For general information about hospice, you can go to *www. cancer.org* and enter "hospice" in the search engine.

∽ You may want to check with your own hospital to learn of hospice organizations in your local area.

## Difficult Conversations about Death and Dying

Conversations about death and dying are never easy, especially when you're immersed in caregiving and focused on your patient's survival, but they often become even more difficult when your patient's condition has deteriorated and the cancer is winning. That's why having these conversations before death is imminent reduces stress on the patient, family members, and friends.

Discussions may include not only the reality of death, but also related issues, such as where to die and at what point to stop treatment. These emotion-laden topics may be raised either by the patient or the caregiver, sometimes in the company of a social worker or other mental health professional. What's important is that they do happen, and preferably sooner rather than later. As long as you are expressing your love and concern for the comfort of the patient and the welfare of those he loves, you may surprise yourself with your ability to set the stage and have the conversation in a manner that is comfortable for everyone involved.

Some families (particularly those who are praying for a miracle) have difficulty confronting the likelihood of death. **Deborah O's husband**, who faced this situation nine months after her diagnosis with Stage 4 inoperable mucinous adenocarcinoma of the lung, has come to realize that for her, saying goodbye may have felt like being unfaithful to the family's hopes and prayers. He suggests in hindsight that:

> *Patients need to be encouraged to say goodbye before they become too ill to do so, even if it turns out to be like the Rolling Stones Farewell Tour which, I think, has been underway since the early 1990s.*

Journals, letters, or even recorded personal messages from the patient to loved ones can offer a permanent record for them to read at key milestones later on. Deborah O's husband realizes now, after her death, how much such messages would have meant to him and their children.

**Doug's mother** offered some helpful tactics for engaging a dying patient in productive dialogue based on the insights and experience she had during her son's last days:

> *One thing I learned not to ask was, "How are you feeling?" but instead to ask, "What are you thinking about?" It provoked some wonderful conversations.*

> *Keep a journal. I kept a separate journal documenting conversations along the way as he was dying, separate from the medical journal.*

> *Doug was on morphine and was lucid till the last day or two. He could interact with his buddies. In fact, they were there so often that parents would apologize if their kid couldn't come. The school waived final exams for four of them. Doug died on the last day of school.*

> *On his final day, before he died, I asked Doug how he wanted to be remembered. I also read comments to him from the notes people had written to him in his yearbook. It was one of the hardest things I had to do, but it was a gift to him.*

Some caregivers engaged the patient in discussions about the process of dying and what legacy they hoped to leave. **Jim D's daughter** was in the difficult situation of having to be the one to tell him that he was dying:

> *The doctor called to explain that the cancer was progressing and they didn't think there was anything further they could do. He asked if I wanted to tell him or preferred to wait for him to get there later that night. I said I'd tell him because I wouldn't be able to be normal all day now that I knew what was happening.*
>
> *It was awful. I remember he sat up in the hospital bed and my mom was beside him. I sat on the floor below them. I said, "The doctor called. It is myelodysplasia, and the only treatment is transfusions. They've never seen anyone transfused so often, but they're willing to do it as long as you want to."*
>
> *We all started crying. He was only 67 years old but said, "I don't want to do it anymore." We said we'd support any decision he made.*

At the time of this writing, **Ellen W's husband** is living with the agonizing uncertainty of not knowing how long his wife will live because her metastasized colon cancer is stage IV. Communicating with her about that is proving difficult:

> *My business partner's son was diagnosed at age three with leukemia and was told he had only three years to live, and he's 21 now. So I've talked with him about how you live with someone who's so precious to you and could die at any time, and how it changes your perspective.*
>
> *Last summer I had to go through these stages of denial, anger, and so on. Now Ellen and I are living life with cancer together, and even though the shock of the cancer coming back this summer was a blow, it was just a reminder of the seriousness of the situation.*
>
> *Probably the most difficult communication is between Ellen and me. She said she knows I'm there for her physically*

*but not always emotionally. Sometimes she has to kick me in the seat of my emotional pants for me to realize that I have somehow pulled away.*

*I went to talk to our social worker about what I can do if Ellen dies. How can I cope as a single parent? How will our daughter handle it? How do you even go through the death of a spouse in the long term with a child? It scares the heck out of me. I needed the chance just to say to our social worker that I fear more for our daughter than for me. I keep thinking that when she's 21, she'll either say to both of us, "Tell me what happened back then," or she'll say to me, "I just really miss Mom."*

The prospect of impending death causes some patients to share stories and feelings that come as news to their caregivers. **John's daughter** found that some of the last conversations with her father before he died of mesothelioma were among the most memorable and meaningful they had ever had:

*Losing someone to a gradual illness is heart-wrenching because you're seeing his strength wither away when before he was larger than life. Yet it was a blessing because we had so many conversations individually and as a family.*

*We talked about things like what did he expect after he died. He defined what he thought he was going to see and experience. Nothing was unspoken between my father and me. He also said, "I'll always be there, but you just won't see me. When the sun is out, it's just me breaking into your world." Sometimes I feel his presence more than others.*

Similarly, **George's daughters** learned a great deal about their family's history during his final days:

*Before he passed, we spent time with him and documented his past and heard stories that we'd misunderstood as kids. We typed them up. It was something we could share later, when we were together. It was a good way to spend our time*

*and gave him something to talk and laugh about. He an-*
*swered lots of our questions.*

Susan was suffering from a glioblastoma brain tumor, and her memory was severely impaired toward the end of her life. Yet her daughters say that there were times when glimpses of her former self re-emerged and allowed for memorable conversations that helped the three of them come to grips with the fact that she was dying. One of **Susan's daughters** remembered:

*When people would come, she'd put on a smile and a wel-*
*coming face. She didn't remember their names, but she called*
*them all "sweetie." One night around 1 a.m., she was lucid.*
*She looked at us and said, "Thank you for letting me be here*
*and taking care of me." Those moments were few and far be-*
*tween. You had to wait for them.*

*Over the summer, there would be short discussions about*
*people who had already passed away. Our biological father*
*had died when we were ages seven and eight. She had been*
*married to our stepfather Don for 26 years. We asked, "Mom,*
*will it feel as though you're cheating on Don when you see*
*Daddy?" She said, "No, it will be like seeing an old friend."*
*Once she realized people she wanted to see again were wait-*
*ing for her, she definitely started to accept her situation.*

While Jim D was dying of myelodysplasia as a result of his treatments for mesothelioma, he made his family promise that he wouldn't be buried before his elderly mother, who was still living. **Jim's daughter** describes their good-byes:

*We brought his 98-year-old mom to say good-bye when he*
*was in the hospital. That was one of the hardest times. He*
*didn't know we were bringing her. We wheeled her into the*
*room, and he said, "Oh, my mama." Almost like a little child*
*would say. They visited, and they both knew. It was really*
*hard for her. She knew he was sick, but didn't know the ex-*
*tent. We hadn't wanted to upset her, but we'd do it again.*

His family saved the urn with Jim's ashes, put it on the altar when his mother died, and placed her ashes into her grave before burying his.

Occasionally a patient will orchestrate his or her own death in a way that starts healing for others even before caregiving is over. When **Stephanie**, a 35-year oncology nurse, was dying of a blood cancer, she and her friends ensured that her young adult son had a safety net of nurses to help answer all of his questions. Then she engaged him in discussion about every aspect of what would come, including how she wanted to be buried (in her full length fur coat and red high heels). Those discussions were poignant, open, and loving, and they brought humor and comfort into his world at just the time he needed them most.

Although conversations like these near the time of death can be heart-wrenching, in retrospect many caregivers felt that they were important and memorable, and that they created a positive sense of closure.

## The Lasting Impact of Unexpected Kindnesses

Several of the caregivers told stories of receiving unanticipated kind gestures shortly before or after loved ones' deaths. For **John's daughter**, who was helping her father through the last stages of mesothelioma, the high school band's acknowledgement of his long-time support warmed her heart and gave the surviving family something to smile about:

> *Dad had been very active in the small town where we grew up. My sisters and I had been in the band, and our parents stayed with the band even after we had all graduated. He would go on their trips and carry the uniforms in his truck.*

> *In June of his last year, the band members knew he was getting sicker because he hadn't gone on a trip that year. The town declared June 12 to be John Davis Day, and the band performed in the yard of our house. The kids visited him, and the selectmen went through all sorts of formalities. Dad sat on the deck with my sisters and close family friends to enjoy it.*

Although **Jim D's daughter** had talked with her dad about his funeral in advance—he had been a firefighter in the town where they lived—she was surprised by the unexpected honor his peers accorded him:

> *I had had the talk with my dad and asked what he wanted for his service. He said, "I'll be dead, I won't care, so whatever makes your mom and you guys happy, do it." My mom wanted to have the services for him as a firefighter.*

> *The firemen all came; they had an honor guard at the wake. On the way, they did a turnout at his fire station. They stopped the hearse and turned the truck in a circle, and they were all lined up out there saluting. Then they marched in formation from the funeral home to the church with bagpipes playing. It was the most beautiful thing I'd ever seen. We went all through town, around a pond, to the church. He was a 30-year veteran, and they wanted to do that for him.*

In the case of Doug, his female **oncologist** at the children's hospital where he spent his last days developed a strong relationship with Doug and the family. She described it with real caring:

> *As Doug was dying, I felt that there was nothing I could do medically, so I brought a litter of kittens to their house. Doug loved them and kept one of them who comforted him in those last days. The family still has the cat.*

> *I remember his last day in the hospital. I had to go to National Guard duty in another town, of all things. At the end of the day, I ran into his room in my combat boots and uniform, hoping to see him, but he had just died. His parents were still at his bedside, and they said Doug would have laughed at me in those boots and uniform.*

**Doug's mom** said that the fact that his oncologist made the effort to try to see him before he died meant more to his family than she could find words to express.

Such gestures as a death approaches or immediately thereafter can become lasting memories that sustain family caregivers long after the event itself.

## Helping a Patient to Die With Dignity

The caregivers who contributed to this book were generous in sharing their stories about how they helped their loved ones to die with dignity and improved comfort. These stories show people at their most noble, courageous, and generous. **Joe's wife** captured the feeling well when she said:

> *The dignity with which people can die, and the legacy they leave, is amazing. There's no right and there's no wrong. Everyone handles it differently.*

This section deals first with facing a terminal diagnosis, managing the expectations of everyone involved, and then with planning the death so it has the maximum positive impact on those left behind. Planning includes choices about when and where to die. All of this may sound unreal to a first-time caregiver. At the start of the cancer journey, you may feel that there's nothing positive about the possibility of your patient dying. Yet the interviewed caregivers indicated that they were better able to cope if their expectations were managed appropriately and that in many cases, the *way* in which a loved one died had a lasting positive impact on their lives and their memories of him.[36]

### Facing a Terminal Diagnosis

When she died sooner than expected after a seven-year battle with appendiceal cancer, **Debbie B's husband** explained how he managed to cope:

> *The kids' helplessness was basically the same as mine. That's a very important part of an acceptance that any caregiver needs to come to grips with. You are actually in someone else's hands.*

---

36 Specific guidance about the dying process and actions caregivers need to take can be found at *www.cancer.net*, the website of the American Society of Clinical Oncology.

*If you're religious, it's God. If you aren't, it's fate. Whatever it is, you're not going to be able to control this cancer or the way your loved one deals with it. It's between them and the disease.*

*You're there to support the person who's battling the disease, but you can't change the outcome. As a patient, Debbie very much wanted to be in control, and for her it was hard to give up. She never gave up—her insides did.*

My neighbor Bill was a public health physician in his 70s who had taught at the college level, held state government office, and traveled extensively through Africa on public health missions. He had been in care for metastasized lung cancer for over a year and thought he'd beaten it. Then, when he was told that he had only months to live, he and his wife went on a farewell tour around the world to visit friends they had made in their previous travels. **Bill** kept a running blog on CaringBridge:

*Jane and I have concluded that this dying business is damn near a full-time job, particularly if you want to have a hand on the wheel of fate. The other evening we said to each other, "Our lives have never been better." We have the time and the opportunity to be with family and friends and to savor the richness of life. Medicine and technology are great, but friends and family are what make every day a pleasure and worth living.*

Even as he faced death, Bill continued to teach others.

In the words of **Nancy's husband**, who has become philosophical about death:

*We all have an expiration date. We can take a million roads to get there, but the date's the date.*

## Managing Expectations

One of the most important elements of the dying process is managing the expectations of both patient and caregiver. **Tim S's wife** reached out to others for that information:

*We had asked the oncologist to tell us what would happen and how. The hospice nurses knew that I was a nurse and wanted to be the one who was doing the primary caregiving. Having her accessible meant that I could ask for help when I needed it.*

*A book they gave us was "Final Gifts." We all read it and all found it useful. There's lots in it about communication between patient and family, even if you can no longer talk but are conscious. The way people communicate when they can't talk can still be loving communication—nodding or making eye contact or moving their lips. We could still communicate even though Tim didn't have the words any more.*

Hospice nurses also point out that the patient's sense of hearing is still functioning as the patient is dying. That realization has proven to be a comforting insight for many of the caregivers who kept their loved ones company during their dying moments.

For **Claire's daughter**, the failure of the medical team to explain what would happen when her mother stopped treatment left a lasting ache in her memories:

*My mother made the decision to have the tubes taken out, and the nurse came in to say it's time to do that. Mom had been intubated for a week and a half and hadn't spoken, so I had hoped that she'd be able to talk to us. I had this vision in my head that they're going to take the tubes out and she's going to wake up and talk to us, but when they took the tubes out and we came back in the room, she never woke up. I really regret that.*

*The nurse did us a great disservice in not telling us what would happen. At the end stages, make them explain to you exactly what's going to happen, because you'll never get those moments back once they're gone.*

**Jeanette**, who has been a serial caregiver for several close friends who died of cancer, knows how important it is for caregivers to understand what can happen when a patient who has fought cancer for some time comes to the end of his journey. Sometimes the patient starts to distance himself from the living as he prepares to die:

> *One coping mechanism for the patients is to pull away from their friends. It's a coping mechanism and a level of acceptance that they're dying. It's hard for the caregiver, who wants to keep fighting and giving, but it represents a gradual acceptance when the patient is just too tired to be with people.*

The most valuable resources in preparing caregivers for the dying process can be hospice professionals and the publications they offer. In addition, there are several resources where end-of-life issues are addressed, including:

- &#x2766; "The Little Blue Book" is available in several forms. One is called "Gone From My Sight," which is available from *www.GoneFromMySight.com*. This version is written by Barbara Karnes, an experienced hospice nurse and trainer.

- &#x2766; "Final Gifts" by Maggie Callanan and Patricia Kelley, Bantam Books, 1993 (Paperback, 239 pages) was cited by several caregivers as having been invaluable.

- &#x2766; The American Cancer Society's website offers helpful information by searching for "hospice" or "end of life."

- &#x2766; The American College of Physicians at *www.acponline.org.*

## Planning for Death

Most of us have a hard time wrapping our heads around the idea of deciding when and where we're going to die. Yet many caregivers who have experienced their patient's death urge new caregivers to learn more about their choices when it becomes clear that the journey's end is near. They agree that the two most important considerations are where the patient is and who is with him when he dies.

A study of whether the location of a patient's death makes a difference to him or his caregiver was published in the "Journal of Clinical Oncology" in September 2010.[37] It was based on interviews with 342 patients and caregivers dealing with advanced cancer. The authors followed the patients from the time of enrollment in the study until they died, for an average of 4.5 months. They evaluated patients' quality of life during their final months and assessed caregivers' mental health both at enrollment in the study and six months after the patient's death. Their key findings were striking:

- ∼ Caregivers of cancer patients who died in intensive care units had a five-fold greater risk of developing Post-Traumatic Stress Disorder (PTSD) compared with caregivers of patients who died at home with hospice services.

- ∼ Patients who died in the hospital experienced more physical and emotional distress and worse quality of life than those who died at home.

- ∼ Caregivers whose patients died in the hospital were four times more likely to experience prolonged grief disorder than those whose patients died at home or in hospice.

The authors of the study attributed the difference to increased dialogue and more education for caregivers about end-of-life care.

Sometimes the option of dying at home is constrained because—as in Debbie B's or Didier's case—the patient's physical condition requires him to be in the hospital, where he can be kept most comfortable. Nowadays, the availability of hospice care in a variety of settings gives patients and their caregivers other options that were not available just a few years ago.

For those who have a choice, the decision often depends on both the patient and those who will be left behind. Some caregivers have been

---

37  "Cancer Advances: News for Patients from ASCO's Journal of Clinical Oncology," September 13, 2010 (*www.cancer.net* and search for "where patients die").

trained by nurses or nurse practitioners to give the patient injections, perform hydration, provide intravenous feeding, and reprogram pumps that deliver medication. Annie's husband even learned to drain fluid build-ups from Annie's lungs, change catheters, and change dressings on abdominal wounds that wouldn't heal.

Such practical training may let the patient experience less travel and stress during a time that is already difficult. According to **Mike S's wife**:

> *It allowed us to be more independent, meaning less time at the hospital and, the greatest gift of all, to be comfortably home and together as a family during his last days.*

Several of the caregivers orchestrated the place of death in ways that created warm and wonderful memories that have kept the patient alive in their minds even years after the event. **Mike S's wife** helped her husband die in a favorite place surrounded by loved ones:

> *When we decided not to return to the hospital, we went to our beach house. Mike wanted to be there. He spent his last day on the couch, looking at the view, seeing the kids come and go. It was very peaceful to have these last moments alone together with just our family. He died at home with us.*
>
> *I was at a workshop once with health care workers discussing end of life. There were many oncology nurses there. The leader asked the participants how they would want to die: hit by a truck, in their sleep, and so on. Many said they would want to die of cancer because you have time to say good-bye and nothing would be left unsaid.*
>
> *Mike embraced life while facing death, and it was inspiring for all of us. Mike's last words were to Anne, our daughter, telling her that he loved her. It was a soul-searing experience to watch someone I loved walk inexorably toward certain death with courage, dignity, and humor.*

**Frank's son**, who was in emotional agony at the prospect of losing his father and best friend, described moving him from a hospice facility so he could die at home in surroundings that he loved:

*They medicated him because of the agitation, which they said was a sign of dying. There was little interaction after that. My older sister said, "We'll get you home." We got him a hospital bed and set him in front of the window overlooking the lake. He wasn't conscious. I said welcome home, and he squeezed my hand.*

*It was 11:00 or 11:30 at night when he died. My sisters were in bed, and I was up with my mom. I went to say good night to him. She said to him, "OK. It's OK. You can let go." Then I said, "Go to God. Just go." About an hour or so later, the dog barked from another part of the house. I woke Mom, and she heard Dad take his last breath. He was still warm. We talked a couple of minutes, and I pulled his eyes shut. He was at peace. Mom and I just sat there with him from 1 a.m. to 5 or so, talking after we tucked him in.*

There's not much more difficult in life than saying good-bye to someone you care about who is dying, and you may feel like avoiding doing so because it can be quite painful. Several of the caregivers, however, talked about the importance of not having regrets. They urge making sure you say everything you want to say to the person before he dies. You can't say it too soon, but if you wait, it might just become too late. Because hearing is the last sense to go, however, you can share an important message even very near the end.

For **Jacqueline's husband**, it was important that all of the children got the opportunity to say good-bye:

*They kept her alive so my sons could come in from Japan to say good-bye. I really appreciated that. Jacqueline wasn't conscious but she wasn't dead. We all talked to her. Everyone got the chance to say good-bye. It was consoling for all of us. I provided all of her care, with no hospice. What was hard was to look at someone you love and realize she's dying. You want to show her how much you love her and to make that transition as comforting as possible and as painless as possible.*

Saying good-bye in written or recorded form is a thoughtful gift that some dying patients provide for the consolation of their loved ones after they are gone. It gives the survivors something they can review and cherish in their low moments. For more guidance on how to say good-bye, *www.caring.com* is a good resource.

Some caregivers described engaging in some of the patient's favorite activities during the dying process. For Tim S, it was watching baseball on television, as **Tim's wife** explained:

> *During the last couple of days, as he was truly dying, it wasn't a very scary time for us. We knew what to expect. We spent time together. We had moved our bed downstairs into a room with a sofa and chair and TV. The kids were all adults. We sat on the bed with him and talked with him during the last couple of days. He was kind of in a coma, but we talked to him. He'd open his eyes but wasn't talking to us or eating.*
>
> *Tim died at about 9 p.m. It was the first day of baseball season. We were all on the bed watching the game, and our son was telling him about the game. We were also playing music he liked. It wasn't at all scary. Someone noticed that his breathing had changed. We sat with him and held him until he stopped breathing. It was incredibly sad, but not scary.*

Artie knew that he was dying. He made that clear to his extended family and alerted his **daughter-in-law** when the end was near:

> *The hospice nurse said that most people die when the person they want to be present is there, or if they want to be alone when they die, they die alone. She said not to stress about it: "Sometimes a clingy child will be hovering, and when he runs out for coffee, then Mom or Dad dies."*
>
> *Thursday morning Artie said, "I'm not doing too well." My whole extended family is extremely close to my father-in-law, and I told him they were coming to see him. He said they'd better not wait too long. So everyone came down and said*

*their good-byes. He was alert enough that they could sit and chat with him.*

*Friday night, a friend who is a nurse stopped in; Artie really adored her. Baseball was on TV, and she went in to say hello. She called out, "Guys, you'd better come in here."*

*We went in and everyone grabbed a beer because we knew that's what he would want, and we toasted the Red Sox. He was conscious, but not talking. We blessed him, and we had a toast for him. Literally within 30 seconds, he took his last breath. He went peacefully.*

Peace, company, and comfort is what many patients seek as they die. **Ellen S's niece** had been a licensed massage therapist working in a chiropractic office when she decided to pursue additional certification in oncology massage, a specialized skill. When her paternal aunt was treated for breast cancer and then diagnosed with cancer in her kidney and bones, Jenny sought to comfort Ellen as she was dying:

*Dying in pain was the one thing that really scared her, so we had always promised her that we wouldn't let that happen. I gave her a gentle massage as she was dying, and I could see her face loosen up and her body soften. It was an honor and has forever changed my life to know that I could make her death more comfortable.*

Even though most of the caregivers didn't have Jenny's professional training, they found it comforting to be at their patient's side at the moment of death. They expressed appreciation for being able to exchange last words and to offer comfort through their presence.

# Chapter Thirteen

# The Aftermath

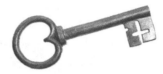

Every cancer journey has an aftermath, and it can last a long time. For patients who "beat" their cancers and for most caregivers, it means returning to a cancer-free life and working to regain a sense of normalcy. For others, the aftershocks may reverberate for decades, especially if their patient didn't survive. Few caregivers I met were able to tell their stories with dry eyes, even if their cancer experiences had occurred decades earlier. They talked candidly about the surprises they faced once cancer treatment was over, as well as how caregiving changed them in fundamental ways.

This chapter shares aftermath stories of five types:

> **Life after the Cancer Crisis**
>
> **The Void After a Patient Dies**
>
> **Grieving and Sources of Comfort**
>
> **Dreams and Visions of Loved Ones Lost**
>
> **Healing as a Deliberate Strategy**

## Life After the Cancer Crisis

Many who experience a life-threatening cancer crisis and go on to live cancer-free feel that they have been given a reprieve, a second chance. While their outlook may have changed in the process, they—like **Richard's wife**—are ready to get on with their lives:

> *I have faith and hope it doesn't come back, but I won't dwell on the possibility. Richard had 10 wonderful years of retirement*

*before he got sick. The doctor is amazed how well he's do-ing. Every three months, Richard goes for treatment with Rituxan. The Rituxan is like a smart bomb: If there are any cancer cells left, it will attack them. It feels like we've had a miracle. He went through it, he fought it, and he's doing well. It may come back, but I'm not worried about it as much now.*

Tiffany and her husband now look back on her cancer experience with a sense of gratitude. Seven years before, at age 33, she was given only a 50% chance of surviving her stage III-c colorectal cancer. That diagnosis and the stress of her cancer treatment changed **Tiffany's husband's** view-point forever:

*The cancer may be physically over, but not mentally. The pos-itive outcome is that we look at life now more on a day-to-day basis. I appreciate what I have. I say, "I love you" more. I have a better appreciation of the need to put things in per-spective and appreciate the little things—family, kids, life in general. It helps you put the stupid things away.*

That realization was the most common reaction of cancer caregiv-ers after the crisis was over: little setbacks and inconveniences no longer mattered.

At the same time, after getting used to the intensity, pace, and adrena-line rush that accompany each health crisis, many caregivers found it hard returning to everyday life. Some—like **Rob's wife**—were conditioned to the flurry of treatment activities:

*Now we're three weeks from being done with Rob's proton beam treatment. All the treatment activity and knowing that we're doing things to help him have been calming. We'll prob-ably fall back into old routines, but I really need to think about what I will change about our life. We have an 80% chance of no recurrence within five years, but I'm fearful of the follow-up MRI. How do you go on without thinking about that?*

**James' wife**, who has dealt with her husband's incurable cancer for over 20 years, has become adept at living with the disease, but she admits that she, too, had problems adjusting at first:

> One of the hardest things was after the first transplant when he was back at work, having set a record on the speed of recovery. I was frantic that we weren't doing anything. I always felt the need for us to be doing something. I was surprised to hit the wall when nothing was going on.

> Cancer in this kind of situation becomes a part of the fabric of your life. Once a week I review all the pills he takes and fill up boxes of pills. Monthly we have blood checks testing for cancer.

> At some point you get philosophical. About a year after the first transplant, he called me at work and said, "I'm fine but your car isn't." A pink Buick had screamed through an intersection and hit him broadside. I got mad at him! I was a crazy person. Then I realized that all we've got is what we've got, and it helped me with my perspective. After all, every one of us has a pink Buick somewhere in our life.

Most caregivers continued to experience a variety of anxieties for a long period during their cancer aftermath. For Tracy, who completed her treatment for non-Hodgkin's lymphoma 20 years ago, fear strikes each time she goes for her annual checkup. A successful internist and cancer prevention physician in an inner city teaching hospital, she is married and has two happy and healthy children. Yet according to **Tracy's husband**, they still experience exam anxiety:

> Her annual checkups always make me jittery. When she's going in for that visit, I say my prayers before I go to bed and when I wake up, and that's all I can do. Even 20 years later, we feel it.

> So there is a back-to-normal. We're back to normal except for that one day each year, and 364 out of 365 isn't bad. When everything is fine, I don't worry about it for another year. You can't, because there's too much else in life.

**Paul's wife** also continues to worry about her husband's health many years later:

> *After his treatments ended, I had anxiety attacks. I couldn't sleep, so I'd leave the bedroom and lie down on sofa cushions on the floor. I kept looking at the clock and couldn't stop my mind from racing. I knew it was a trauma from the cancer experience.*
>
> *Things never get back to normal. Even though we're coming up on the 13-year anniversary of his diagnosis, it never goes completely away. Anxiety remains. We both knock on wood whenever we bring it up.*

Judy M finished her treatments for metastatic breast cancer over 10 years ago, but twice when she experienced unexpected physical symptoms, she and her husband found their rational and emotional selves engaged in a tug-of-war. **Judy M's husband** said:

> *We hadn't been down this path before, so we had no frame of reference. Before her diagnosis, we had no reason to be really frightened, but now, when an unexpected symptom arises, it pushes all of those buttons of fear, anxiety, and uncertainty. It raises mortality concerns. She's extremely cognizant and proactive about her checkups. Yet it's always in the back of our minds.*

In contrast to these caregivers, whose patients are cancer-free, **Tom's wife** is living with ongoing uncertainty about the status of her husband's rare retroperitoneal liposarcoma, which created an eight-pound tumor in his abdomen:

> *It takes a while to realize that for most things, you go to the doctor to fix it, but some things aren't totally fixable. As much as you may like and trust your doctors, it's an art being a doctor, and it's not all fixable. Confronting the fact that you never know how things are going is hard.*
>
> *Tom's cancer may keep coming back because they never know whether they've gotten it all. You have to plan to live and whatever happens, happens.*

Michael S is living with incurable cancer, so the aftermath for his family is like living under a dark cloud that won't go away. As **Michael S's father** explains:

*This March will represent 10 years for him. Our life is now a new normal. We cannot remember life before cancer. It has changed the journey that we thought we were on. Our daughter is the only member of the immediate family who hasn't had cancer. As a result, our perspective has changed significantly. We have friends who talk long-term about their kids—what they'll do professionally, when they'll buy a house, get married, and so on. We focus on today.*

*Michael still lives at home. He works 30 hours a week, and of the three bosses that he has had so far, two are cancer survivors, so it really helps give him support. It also helps that he is protected against job discrimination by the Americans with Disabilities Act and the Family Medical Leave Act.*

*Three years ago, they discovered a couple of new tumors in his liver and spine. They are inoperable, and they don't respond to radiation or chemotherapy at the cellular level. He is now in a clinical trial to keep the cancer in check, and there is some shrinkage.*

*I was at a training session at work that was also a team-building exercise. We were asked to draw a picture of our life story. It was hard for me because I couldn't remember life before cancer. The cancer experience stays as a raw wound. We have a strong family support system, but lots of us have had cancer—myself, my wife, my son, both of my in-laws, and my wife's sister. I found the exercise very upsetting.*

*Every doctor's visit, even though the cancer is static, triggers anxiety and fear. Our daughter is married and has a future. Our son has a job but maybe no future. We stay in the moment and just don't plan ahead.*

When Jacqueline was dying, she remained adamant that she wanted her husband to find a female companion. Even though he didn't deliberately set out to date after Jacqueline's death, serendipity struck, and he found a wonderful woman who fills part of the hole that Jacqueline left behind. More challenging than the conversation with Jacqueline before she died was his discussion with their children after he decided he wanted to marry again. When asked how he managed to retain the love he had had for his wife while learning to love someone else again, **Jacqueline's husband** replied:

> *I came to realize that it's like the love you have for your children. You love each of them individually and for who they are. I loved each of them for different reasons. You don't love one more than the other. I told them that if you understand that concept, you'll understand why I want to marry again.*
>
> *The kids gave me a rough time. My current wife helped me so much going through that process, because my attitude was "who the hell are they to tell me what to do with my life?" She said, "Wait a minute, don't you want to have them in your life? You can't ram me down their throats."*
>
> *It took a good three years to win them over. They had a very difficult time seeing me with another woman. Before we got married two years ago, I went to Japan and personally asked my sons to come to the wedding. They did, but I know it had to hurt them.*
>
> *We talked about that. "Here's the thing you have to remember," I said. "I loved your mother very much, and I went out of my way to do everything I could for her. The good Lord took her, and there's nothing I could do about that. She wanted me to be happy. I can't live alone. I need someone to talk to. Someone to have dinner with. Someone to cook for."*

Most of the caregivers who were interviewed felt that it is essential not to let the cancer aftermath stop you from living, regardless of what worries and fears linger. They recommended that you acknowledge your anxiety about relapses, so you can recognize when it happens and then put it away.

They also urge focusing on today and on the joys that remain in life, rather than the things that cancer has taken away.

## The Void after a Patient Dies

When someone you cared for dies, it feels like a hole has developed in your life that may never be filled. Most of us are sad about such a loss, but for caregivers, the grief is likely to be more intense. Learning to get beyond the constant sense of emptiness may seem like an overwhelming task.

While everyone grieves differently, interviewees suggested some things to do that can help ease the caregiver's pain and sense of loss after the patient dies:

- ❧ Reaching out to other caregivers who have shared a similar experience may make you feel less alone.

- ❧ Writing down stories of good times that might have been shared in the patient's final days gives something tangible and positive to recall when you're feeling most alone. **Doug's mom** and **George's daughters** found this to be helpful.

- ❧ Keeping a journal of your feelings and experiences may help you get a grip on them. You may also feel that you're sharing them, if only by writing them down.

- ❧ Communicating with the patient's closest friends and sharing how much the patient cared about them is a way to maintain contact and build new bonds. **Carole's husband** valued such ongoing connections.

- ❧ Anticipating rituals, anniversaries, and other events that draw attention to your loved one's absence can help spur you to make alternative plans. Spending the time with other people can partially fill the sense of emptiness and distract you with something pleasant. **Nick's parents** now spend the Christmas holidays across the country, with their daughter.

For **Debbie B's husband**, the void felt virtually overwhelming two months after her sudden death, and it became almost palpable during the interview. He started the conversation sounding strong, but before long he couldn't hold back his tears:

> One of the things I've experienced is that for years I was very much involved in fighting cancer with her. But then she died. It's all over. There's no fight any more, and we lost. The absence of something to fight against or push against is a real problem for me. During caregiving, your life really does center around the disease. I expected to have more time to adjust to the fact that she wasn't going to be here.

> It's confusing, because I'm still so deep in the grieving process. I'm bitter. I didn't used to have the feeling "Why us?" and "Why me?" Now it's a cosmic feeling, and I have no target for it.

> I'm much more serious than in the past. So much of my life has changed. I retired from a job I had for 27 years where I was an integral part of important people's lives, and I'm not any more. I used to talk all day with people, and now I talk to nobody. We sold the house we'd lived in for 27 years and moved. And I've lost my spouse, so I'm having to redefine everything in my life.

> I'm a little scared about what my life will be like in five years, and what do I do now? This is a tough time. Someone asked recently, "What do you do all day?" It's like they don't know what else to say. I don't have the desire to do anything right now. I'm just trying to get through the day.

**Sharon's sister** also experiences the absence of the fight, which ended over three years ago. She's now being forced to confront the void Sharon's death has left in her life:

> I thought that focusing on tasks would protect me from being overwhelmed. I was grateful she wasn't suffering any more. I thought I'd process this and get through it. But it's three years now and something will happen that makes me realize she's

*the only person I'd call on this, and I can't. It never goes away. I wanted it to stop for her sake, but it will never stop for me.*

*I think, "You're not here. I want to talk with you right now." Cognitively you say you'll be OK with that, but you're not. The rational part had helped me. It gave me things to do. I told myself I'll just get used to not having a sister. But you don't.*

*That's what I'd like to prepare someone for. You can be the best caregiver ever and the best forecaster of what needs to be done and the best organizer ever, but you can't keep the emotion away. I thought I could keep it away if I had a plan and was organized. I thought it wouldn't affect me so much, but it comes and goes. I thought I'd process this and get through it, but it's been three years now and it hasn't gone away.*

**Annie's husband** experienced almost the same reaction, initially focusing on things that had to be done, and then suddenly having to confront the hole. He reached out to me less than three weeks after Annie's death. When I called him back to set up the appointment and asked how he was doing, he shared that he was lonely and lost, but eager to talk:

*The reality is that I was really busy after Annie died, but I'm totally lost right now. I don't know what to do with myself. I call myself the lost ball in the high weeds. I'm totally lost and lonesome and hurting. I know I'm never going to get over this, but I hope the pain diminishes.*

**Artie's daughter-in-law** had a very similar experience after Artie died:

*I remember those first days, like the week when you're planning the funeral, and then you have the funeral, and people are stopping by with all this food. About a week later, we said, "What do we do?" We felt like we had nothing to do, even though we still had the same busy lives.*

*I was so unbelievably lonely because I work from home and I'd had someone to talk to every day. I could chat and be working at the same time. All of a sudden the house was*

231

*empty, peaceful, quiet. But obviously you're also walking around with your heart broken and terribly sad. You pick up the salt shaker and think, "Oh, I just filled that up for Artie last week." Everything reminds you.*

For **Chuck and Laura's brother**, serial caregiving and losing two siblings had left him with a number of additional relatives in need of care. It made processing his own grief and dealing with the holes left in his own life even more challenging:

*You need to learn to compartmentalize parts of your life. After Chuck died, I said to myself that I needed to figure out how to sleep so I could care for our parents and my sister. It was indescribable, caring for our parents, my brother-in-law, Chuck's wife, their daughter, and my own family. I couldn't complain because I was still standing and had to care for them all.*

*My brother's wake and funeral was gut-wrenching. The reception after the funeral was very long. Everyone in town had to give their condolences. The next morning, I woke up, and I looked out the window and saw the cars were still moving and people were still going to work. I thought, "How can people still be going through normal life when my life will never be the same?"*

*With my sister's death, the hole was no smaller, and the grief was no less. But the second time, you know that life goes on. If you don't go on, then you're no good to anyone. Our mom had her innards ripped out twice. A couple of times she would give me a crack in the head and say things that really stuck: "You know, the hole never gets any smaller. If you don't become a bigger person around it, how do you think you could get out of bed in the morning? If you ever have a question about what's the right thing to do, just remember it's generally the hard thing."*

The hole left by the loss of a loved one seems to be permanent, and most caregivers whose patient had died were still learning to cope with that. But there is often an additional challenge. Several of the caregivers described changes on the part of their friends who had been supportive during the cancer battle:

> **Didier's wife**  *Before, everyone put their arms around me, but afterward they went away. You wear them out because you need so much support. No one wants to hear it. Even my parents don't know what to say.*

> **Carole's husband**  *Carole had lots of friends. For the first few years, they were there. This is the first year that on the anniversary of her death, there were very very few people who got in touch with me again. As more time goes by, it really is out of sight, out of mind. Maybe it's the wrong expectation that friends would remember.*

> **Tim N's wife**  *After Tim died, that's when I felt really alone. Everyone leaves and goes back to their lives, and you're left ravaged. Three years of a disrupted and crazy life with lots of people around. Then the person dies, and after a very short period of time, you're alone. Four years later, I don't find many people who are actually willing to talk about it anymore.*

Many of the caregivers were surprised how long they felt the need for support, for someone to listen. **John's daughter** suggested that over time, the hole becomes more obvious to you, but other people's expectations about your grief change:

> *The first year, you're still in shock and survival mode. You're simply slugging along, getting through every milestone. In the second year, the reality sets in. It's not that people forgot, but they don't expect you to cry at the drop of a hat anymore.*

> *You also need to respect that each family member is coming from a different perspective. My sister with kids would say, "Aren't you the lucky one that you had time with him and didn't have to worry about taking care of kids?" That was hard to hear, especially when there were times when I was hitting bottom and wished she could have done more. You just have to share your reality and be patient with each other.*

Two of the caregivers found that an empty house and blank schedule exaggerated their awareness of the void. According to **Joe's wife**, who had cared for him for years:

> When Joe died, it was at a time when my nest was becoming empty. I went from a house full to a house empty, and that was very hard. I was alone weeknights because my younger son Matthew started college after a few months. I worked 12-hour days during the week.
>
> The hardest time was on Saturday nights. There was a couple we'd gone to high school with—we'd been friends for 40 years —and we would usually go out to dinner or play cards with them on weekends. So after Joe died, Saturday night was my difficult time.
>
> For a while I'd go out and buy things on Saturday night, not because I needed them, but to get out of the house. I knew what I was doing, and at first I didn't care. After a while I said to myself that Saturday comes around every seven days, and I'll have to learn to deal with it.

Joe's wife is back to work and coping, but she still struggles with how to fill that hole.

**Tim S's wife** had a similar emotional reaction but has taken deliberate action to restore her joy in living:

> I had decided I wanted to stay in our house. We had built it on the family farm, and I knew I was going to stay there. But coming home after work to an empty house was just excruciating.
>
> On the last day that I worked, after the going-away parties, I came home and was alone. It was horrible. Awful. Being home alone that Friday night without having made a plan for it was a very bad idea. It took a little bit to realize it.
>
> Now I do lots of volunteer work at the cancer center. I'm a trustee of the local school where Tim and I taught and where our kids went. I'm a justice of the peace, and I spend time volunteering and traveling. I bought an RV. Two years after

*Tim died, I took a trip around the country. We had talked about doing it to visit friends when we retired, and I realized I could still do that. It was a wonderful trip.*

Tim's wife is filling her life again, doing different kinds of things than she did before, so her new activities and busy schedule are helping to temper the emptiness left by his absence.

## Grieving and Sources of Comfort

Don't be surprised if you find that your pain over the loss of a friend or loved one is hiding just beneath the surface, even years after the patient died. In fact, even in cases in which the patient has recovered and is doing well, some caregivers experience grief for the loss of normalcy. They describe it as being like a demon hiding in a dark closet, erupting when they least expect it, often with an intensity that takes their breath away.

**Jack's daughter** described that aspect of her experience with some irony:

> *Cancer is the gift that keeps giving; the after-effects last for years. I never dealt before with the emotional part of it, so it still comes out when I least expect it. Everyone deals with it differently, but you have to do whatever will keep you from having regrets.*

Samantha beat her childhood leukemia and is thriving today, but **Samantha's mother** still finds that:

> *Years later, after we lived through this, there would be times I'd cry apropos of nothing, and I'd wonder why. Then I'd realize that yesterday or the day before something triggered a memory of Sam's leukemia, so this wasn't about what happened yesterday—it was about the recollection of cancer. You never fully process everything at the time, but you learn to cope. You're coping so much that you're not reflecting on the impact until years later and it comes back in different ways.*

*Afterwards, you never feel that lightness of being when the world was your oyster and you felt like you could do anything. After our leukemia experience, you realize life is a gift. It can leave as quickly as it comes. You need to live your life as if you're going to wake up tomorrow morning and the next morning and your family will be there. But you realize that out there lurking are things you can't control, so you need to just do your best.*

*If, for example, Sam were to relapse or one of us were to get sick for the first time, you've been there. You'll never be as afraid again. You'll never have as steep a learning curve as you did the first time. It doesn't mean you won't grieve life's other tragedies or take them as real setbacks, but you have to realize that the situation will never be that bad again. This could make you very afraid to live. Doing that would be a tragedy.*

For **Nora and George's daughter**, the challenge was the duration of her grief—how long it took her to process the loss of her parents, even though her mother died more than 15 years before her father:

*The biggest frustration was that I thought, "I'll get through this in two or three months. In two or three months I'll be able to navigate my emotions and feelings." I thought I'd be the same person I was before. That's very naïve.*

*The reality is that it takes many many many years. That's one of the key things to learn, that the mourning continues and you grow because of the experience. The mourning never ends.*

Nonetheless, three caregivers who were interviewed soon after the deaths of their patients and others who had experienced a death years before described receiving comfort early on that helped them begin to heal during the grieving process:

**Annie's husband** *Hope Lodge was a godsend to me. It was so close to the hospital. I could stay with Annie as long* *as I wanted to and could have a place nearby to go to sleep. The staff have big hearts. Everything there was spontaneous, and the hugs were real.*

**Tim S's wife** *The people around me were angels who just cared for me and cared for us. We were living on the family farm. My sister-in-law had come home to live there, and having her with Tim's parents and with us was wonderful. I can't imagine what we would have done without that. Imagine watching your oldest son die. It had to be horrible for his parents. I didn't have the energy to take care of them, but she did.*

**Lynn's husband** *We had received lots of support while she was sick, but another revelation was the night of the wake. People kept coming and coming, people I worked with 25 years ago came. 450 people in three hours. The line was wrapped around the building and down the street. It was so comforting to have old friends show up. I'll make an effort in the future not to miss a wake. People were holding me up when I just wanted to fall on the floor.*

For **Jada**, an artist and poet, healing came through creative expression. After her father's death from pancreatic cancer, she started to write poetry to further explore her relationship with him and keep his memory fresh. She now hosts a memorial exhibit in his honor of paintings and multi-media pieces that incorporate poems she created. His presence lives on through her work and brings her comfort.

Part of the healing process is being willing to acknowledge that you did your best, regardless of the outcome. That's hardest for caregivers whose loved ones died. Remember, you were enlisted to help someone through an unpredictable journey, not to change the outcome. Your best is all you can expect to have done.

**Jim G's wife** described herself as a "failed caregiver" because the love of her life died, even though her caregiving had kept him alive for 9 years in the face of a terminal lymphoma diagnosis. Although that was a great achievement, 7 years later she still feels as if she should have done better, even in the face of insurmountable odds. To her, the glass feels more than half empty.

In contrast, **Mike's wife** helped keep her husband alive for 27 months when he was diagnosed with stage 4 pancreatic cancer, despite a 6-week prognosis. More than 13 years later, she considers his additional months of quality life with his family as a victory. She helped create joy every day, even at the end when he died at home without pain or anxiety, so her glass is more than half full today.

There are a number of resources that can help both in dealing with grief and in figuring out how to redeploy the energy that was going into the cancer fight:

᧬ The National Cancer Institute, also part of the NIH, offers support at *www.cancer.gov/cancertopics*. This website is fairly comprehensive and describes various stages of grief, beginning at the point where a patient's death is anticipated. Try "bereavement" in the search engine.

᧬ The U.S. Library of Medicine, part of the National Institutes of Health (NIH), supports a website dedicated to helping people understand and deal with their feelings of grief. Go to *www.nlm.nih.gov* and enter "bereavement" in the search engine.

᧬ Elisabeth Kübler-Ross is famous for her work on death and dying. A summary of her work and her available books can be found at *www.grief.com*. On the same website, David Kessler addresses practical issues, like how to handle holidays after a loved one's death.

᧬ For those whose grief is becoming debilitating, the Mayo Clinic offers help at *www.mayoclinic.com*. Type "complicated grief" into the search engine.

## Dreams and Visions of Loved Ones Lost

Perhaps the most unexpected phenomenon described by caregivers was the fact that they had dreams and visions in which the deceased patient appeared as though he were still alive. It can be shocking when it happens, and most of the people interviewed hadn't ever revealed them to others before:

**Joe's wife** *I had dreams so wonderful that I hated to see them end. He's healthy in them.*

**Sharon's sister** *I've had dreams two or three times where she was alive. She was healthy and happy. My dreams have been when she's healthy, always walking and smiling.*

**June's best friend** *June's death was vicious, miserable. I prayed for her to die. It took two weeks. Last year, one morning, I was just waking up, and I saw her at the foot of my bed. I recognized her dress. She looked at me and said, "I'm fine, don't worry." It made a difference for me in how I mourn for her now. Now I don't think of the pain, but of the funny things we did together over the years. I missed June so much that my heart had a lump in it, but after she visited me, it eased up.*

**Tim N's wife** *I had lots of dreams about him, and they were comforting. In my dreams of him, he's always healthy. I never think of him as being sick any more. My dreams came soon after he died and were so comforting. I really felt his presence for a long time. My older daughter feels that the leaves that are moving outside her window are her father talking to her when they wave in the wind.*

**Frank's son** had a series of inexplicable and almost supernatural experiences that gave additional impact and symbolism to his father's death:

*The next morning after he died, there was a spectacular sunrise. Dad was a flower guy, a sunrise guy, a sunset guy. My sister is a professional photographer and was taking a picture. She asked me to come and look at the results. "Isn't the moon pretty?" she asked.*

*But the moon wasn't out. It was a white spot on a picture. The primary one looked like the moon, but white spots were everywhere. My niece looked at the picture a day later, and she said the largest one was an angel orb and that the other white spots were other people's spirits coming to greet him.*

*Ten days before he died, we were looking out the window and he saw a bald eagle. He saw it, but I didn't. He said, "You'll see it." After he died, the whole family took one last run around the lake in our boat, and there was the eagle. We had gone there for years and had never seen an eagle before."*

**Claire's daughter** only dreamed about her mother once, but she met a medium who said some things that were stunningly accurate:

*I didn't used to believe in mediums and all that. There's a woman whom I've gone to see several times. The things she said were unbelievably spot on. She knows things that no one else knows about my mother.*

*No one knew I'd slept in her bed for a week. She said that my mother appreciated my staying with her. She said my mom was holding a baby. I had a brother that died of Sudden Infant Death Syndrome before I was born that my friends didn't even know about. She talked a lot about dreams, and she believes that when weird things happen, like a light going off, it's part of the spiritual world.*

**Lanie's mother** also had an experience with a medium, someone she had never met before:

*I went to a medium who said, "I see a child on your right shoulder. She has long brown curly hair. She has one green eye and one brown eye. She wants you to not be so sad. She's OK. Her scars are gone. She died with a brain tumor." How could this woman who lived an hour away and never met me before have known that? I'd told her nothing.*

Even if you don't believe in an afterlife, dreams and visions from mediums that appear to bring your loved one back to life serve an important healing purpose. They can be disconcerting at first, largely because so few people talk about them (for fear of how others will react). Each of the caregivers who shared such a story called attention to the fact that their loved one in the dream or vision was healthy again and gave them reassurance or good advice for life ahead. They looked back at their metaphysical experiences with fondness and appreciation for having had one more opportunity to see the patient again in full health. They also appreciated that these "encounters" gave their loved one's death further meaning and closure.

## Healing as a Deliberate Strategy

All caregivers need rejuvenating experiences, regardless of the outcome. Several caregivers who had lost loved ones took spontaneous, unplanned road trips to rediscover sides of themselves that they had neglected during caregiving. Others traveled together with their former patient, combining planned visits to friends throughout the country with unstructured stopovers in new locations. Still others engaged in activities outside their normal prior experiences; discovering new interests reignited their joy in being alive. Advocacy gave some a sense of meaning (see Chapter Fourteen).

Sometimes the process of healing forces you to re-examine your whole life. **Didier's wife** had been a corporate executive and the family's primary wage-earner; Didier had been a stay-at-home dad. When he became terminal, they talked about what she would do, including how she would care for their children. Ten days after his death, she found herself an overwhelmed and impoverished single mother responsible for a four-year-old daughter and a newborn son.

One of her most powerful healing acts was to repeat his funeral service three years later and to bury the notebook in which she had recorded all of his instructions, including his request that she not relocate so as to avoid further unsettling the children. That ritual letting go allowed her to take charge of her own life again. Now, after six years as a full-time mother, she is excited as she  plans to move and re-enter the corporate world. She also  understands that relocating will actually help the children. The values she and Didier shared are still important to her, but her self-confidence is back, together with a zest for life and an appreciation for her own needs for professional fulfillment. She is joyful at having rediscovered herself and says that she didn't realize until recently that she had literally lost herself during her caregiving. There is even a new man in her life who loves her and her children.

Healing takes time, and it requires a purposeful changing of gears, as it is essential to redefining meaning in your own life. In the words of **Tim N's widow:**

> I'm surprised to say that I'm getting remarried. It's been seven years since Tim died. I'll never stop loving him, but I never thought I'd be this happy again."

Rabindranath Tagore, an Indian poet, once wrote: "Clouds come floating into my life, no longer to carry rain or usher storm, but to add color to my sunset sky." His words apply well to most cancer family caregivers, too. Despite the wear and tear they sustained during their difficult journey, as they heal, they may find their life enriched by what they have experienced and learned.

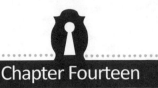

# Chapter Fourteen

# How Cancer Changes Caregivers

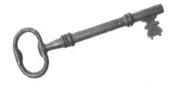

The formal interviews and informal conversations with caregivers and patients revealed that it's nearly impossible to go through a cancer caregiving experience without being changed by it in some meaningful way. The life-and-death implications of a cancer fight, the unpredictability of the caregiver's path, and the somewhat isolating impact of the disease pose the greatest challenges for caregivers. At the same time, they provoke the most profound changes in people.

These changes tended to fall into three categories:

**Discovering Inner Strength**

**Giving Back Through Compassion and Service**

**Returning to Life Without Dark Clouds**

## Discovering Inner Strength

Many of the caregivers with whom I spoke found the caregiving experience surprisingly affirming. They said it had toughened them, deepened their inner resources, and demonstrated their stamina beyond their own expectations about whether they could sustain the level of effort required and navigate the many challenges they faced:

**Mike S's wife**  *I am lonelier but stronger after this experience. I know that no matter how much love and support one has, illness and death happen to only one person, the patient and not the caregiver. I will never say to myself, "I can't do this," because I learned that I can.*

**Tim S's wife**  *I certainly learned that I could do whatever was needed to be done to take care of Tim, and that's what I wanted to do.*

**Ed's wife**  *I think I'm older and wiser now. I'm more patient than I was. You don't sweat the small stuff when you're worried about life and death. As Ed was dying, his eyes opened wide and he got a beautiful look on his face as though he'd seen the light. I'm not afraid of dying, but I'm afraid of losing someone else again.*

**George's daughter**  *When you go through something as difficult as this, you kind of feel you can get through anything emotionally. Nothing since has been that painful or felt more overwhelming. You realize you'll accomplish many things in your life and won't be able to share them with that parent, so the feeling of loss keeps going. Losing a parent at a young age fundamentally changed how I prioritize things.*

Judy M's husband is a recovering alcoholic. He found Judy, the love of his life, after his children were grown. While he was going through a prolonged and difficult divorce, Judy was diagnosed with metastasized breast cancer, and he became her primary caregiver. During her year of treatment she suffered severe reactions to her chemotherapy, resulting in many "lost" weekends. For **Judy M's husband**:

> *Judy's experience was truly life-changing. It was more profound than my own recovery as an alcoholic because this was a life-and-death issue. It was like going through a dark tunnel with the person you're closest with.*

The experience has allowed him to acknowledge and give voice to his feelings more than he was ever inclined to do in his earlier life.

Finally, **Susan's daughters** found helping their mother die to be both fulfilling and affirming:

> *We've done the hardest thing we've ever had to do, and we won't ever have to do it again. The only thing worse would be if something were to happen to one of us. For us, we were there 24/7 loving her, and we got her to where she needed to be. We did that for her. That's comforting. She brought us in, and we helped her go out. We held her hand and said we're OK and you can go, and we'll see you again. For me, that was really important. Some days I'm right back in that room again.*

## Giving Back Through Compassion and Service

Many caregivers found that their experiences with cancer increased their compassion for others facing similar challenges, and they used the life lessons they had acquired in a variety of ways to offer support.

**Annie's husband** found that his experience of literally providing all of the care as his wife battled ovarian cancer gave him a new perspective on himself:

> *What came out of that first go-around for me was learning patience. I had been a very impatient man. If I had something to do, I'd want to get it done right now; I didn't want to mess around. I had absolutely no pain level, so I didn't think anybody else did either. I was just probably like a charging bull. But I learned to slow down, and I learned to have patience. I learned to have some sympathy—to put myself in other people's moccasins for a little while, and to think how I'd like to be treated if I was in their shoes.*

He hopes to apply the knowledge he has acquired in training other caregivers or paramedics.

For some caregivers, like **Tommy's sister**, getting involved in a cause to fight cancer with others who have similar values and a commitment to stop cancer in its tracks is a source of comfort:

*I do the American Cancer Society's Relay For Life each year so I won't have to see another sibling go through what he did. Every year on Tommy's birthday, I go to the cemetery and leave roses.*

**Susan's daughters, Stacey and Kim,** found that returning to day-to-day living after caring for their mother led to an unexpected challenge and opportunity for giving back:

*How do you withdraw from it in the aftermath? It takes a long time. For me, having spent almost two years out of the corporate working world, I needed to get a job. When you're in life and death situations, and then go back to work where people are worried about a schedule deadline, it's like, "Are you kidding me?" I was working, but the work had no real meaning.*

*We'd never heard of or known about brain tumors before Mom got sick. And then what happens? We went on vacation after she died, and we met this little boy who had a brain tumor. We stayed in touch with him and his family and went to his funeral in Baltimore. Then the following winter, our neighbor Jen P had a grand mal seizure and was diagnosed with a brain tumor. Two months later, another friend is in the hospital with a brain tumor.*

*So it seems we're in this brain tumor community, not to leave it again. This is what we do now, raising money and awareness to fight brain tumors.*

Jen P and her husband now collaborate with Susan's daughters to raise money to support the cancer services that were so helpful to both of their families during their respective cancer journeys. As **Jen P's husband** said:

*We've turned this horrible thing that's affected us into a charity to help others in the local area. A lot of our healing has been helping others and keeping the memory of Stacey's mom alive. We also help refer people where to go for help.*

Now that her son is several years beyond his lymphoma treatment, **Jeff's mother** has focused her energies on helping other families who experience childhood cancer. She also spends time advocating for legislative support to increase cancer research funding through ACS's Cancer Action Network. She reflected on how she had changed:

> *I've become more patient with myself; more patient with people who are sick. Life can change in an instant. The experience I shared with Jeff has made me a more giving and forgiving person. It made me appreciate the fact that I get out of bed every day and have the chance to do something about my situation, whether it's good or bad. Every day I try to do something that will either help myself or help someone I care about, and maybe even a complete stranger.*

**Doug's mother** has found ways to give back that are consistent with how Doug wanted to be remembered. She has gotten involved with the National Childhood Cancer Foundation and volunteers with the ACS in the areas of childhood cancers, chemotherapy, and pain control:

> *I'm very different. I'm more accommodating of others' attitudes and behaviors. When people are in a painful place, because of personal and medical situations, I can see it. I get pissed when people are agitated by unimportant things. Your life can be upended, so what are you going to do with it?*
>
> *After Doug died, we started a program for children with cancer at his hospital (a regional children's specialty hospital), as he had requested. His buddies and other kids applied and joined Team Doug to help other kids with cancer there.*

**Michael L's mother** is now on the other side of her son's cancer and feels that his renewed health was a powerful gift. She reflected on how the experience changed her:

> *I'm more cautious now and don't take risks. I feel the rug was ripped out from under me. I'll never forget it as long as I'm breathing.*

Despite living with that fear, she dedicates significant energy to helping other families through the Childhood Brain Tumor Foundation (CBTF):

> *Michael is a sign of hope for others. Michael is walking hope, light at the end of the tunnel. I became a parent-to-parent mentor for the CBTF because of what another mother did for me. It's important to show parents that other parents understand what they're going through.*

Some of the caregiver interviewees were still healing and not yet ready to give back, but many are seeking ways to convert the energy they marshaled during their cancer caregiving to activities that will help others in their battles with the disease. The fact that they took the time to share their experiences in these interviews is another sign of their desire and readiness to "give back" and to try to illuminate caregiving's uncertain path for others.

## Returning to Life without Dark Clouds

The return to living, sometimes *with* cancer, poses challenges that caregivers handle differently, depending on their unique family's situations. Even in the face of a fairly dire prognosis, some caregivers and their patients go on and commit to live life to the fullest.

**Jenn S's husband** is grateful for his wife's current strength and cherishes every day:

> *I'm 36 and still traveling. I'm the envy of some of the guys because I'm going to the Bahamas and they're going to PTA meetings. You have to strike a fine line, at least to us. You don't give up and say, "I'm going to make up a bucket list because I've only got a year." You can't ignore the fact that you know you might not be here in 10 years, so you want to move that trip to Italy up sooner.*
>
> *We've worked really hard at finding a middle ground. Jenn is the only stage IV patient in her support group who's still working, let alone working good hours in a serious career.*

*We don't want to be that couple that just waits for her to die. We've always been ones who focus heavily on traveling and seeing friends and family and doing what we wanted to do. We definitely have a carefree lifestyle that lots of people in our situation wouldn't choose.*

Finally, there are those caregivers like **Sarah**, the nanny who became Ellie and Amy's surrogate mom. As a melanoma survivor, she finds that the caregiving experience causes her to reflect differently on her own experiences with cancer:

*This experience has let me own up to saying "I'm a survivor." My own cancer was really bad at the beginning. Most treatments don't work for melanoma. Caring for the girls and my own cancer journey have made me stronger. The experiences have made me realize that having everything isn't worth it if you're not happy. I'm happy with what I do, even though it's exhausting. I wouldn't trade my life for anything. You could offer me a job with the biggest paycheck, and I'd turn it down.*

*I'm still a wreck around the times of my regular checkups. I do want to have my own kids, but pregnancy can reactivate melanoma, so we'll see what my own doctors say. I've done a lot of good. I hope good karma comes around.*

Sarah's yearning for good karma is a powerful message for all caregivers. After the experiences they go through on their cancer journey, they deserve all the best that life has to offer. But most of all, they deserve the peace of mind that comes from knowing that they gave the fight all they had, and then some.

As they begin to rebuild their lives, deal with loss and the inevitable void it leaves, enjoy a second chance with their loved ones, or continue to battle with and for their patients' health and well-being, many are finding ways to sustain their commitment through involvement in non-profit fund-raising and advocacy efforts. Others are immersed in the challenging process of recovering some sense of personal equilibrium, but all know that life goes on for them, no matter the outcome of their cancer caregiving experiences. Some, like Didier's and Tim N's wives and Doug's mom, are even happy again. Their loved ones are still with them every day, but they've opened the door to new kinds of happiness and live full lives.

# Closing Thoughts

The formal interviews and informal conversations on which this book is based were moving, inspiring, and memorable. No one knows how many of the caregivers' loved ones will survive, or for how long, but it's clear that all of the caregivers felt like survivors of an intense battle. All are moving forward, determined to keep their eyes on the blessings they still have. Their caregiving was a gift to patients who were their family members or close friends. Each of them did his best to ease the experience and achieve a positive conclusion, even if the conclusion was helping the patient to die in comfort and at peace.

Regardless of the outcome, all said that caregiving enriched their lives immeasurably. None of these caregivers' lives will ever be the same. They're stronger, wiser, and more self-confident than when they started their cancer journey. They've already been down the paths that you've begun to walk. Their stories represent their gifts to you, in the hope that they can help you have a smoother trip than they had. Without exception, they were thrilled that their stories still mattered and that the lessons they learned might help you, as a new caregiver.

The lessons these caregivers have shared can increase your range of ideas and approaches going into the experience so you'll feel a little more confident in making your own choices and decisions. In the end, cancer caregiving is about making your own way, so the more tools and alternative ideas you can access, the easier your journey will be.

The stories I've shared are evidence that however tough their trip, the caregivers made it through, and you can do so as well. You didn't ask for the chance to demonstrate your strength, or your caring, or your persistence. The need just landed in your lap. It was fate, or—as Sarah suggested—karma.

Just the fact that you've read this book demonstrates that you have at least some of the persistence necessary to make it through this trip. You're bound to have misgivings along the way, but hopefully these stories will help you overcome self-doubt and second guessing, and encourage you to believe in your ability to perform superbly as a caregiver. Once you get through and have the chance to look back, the odds are good that you'll find you've been as strong as they were.

The caregivers and survivors I interviewed are my friends and my heroes. Many of them have been to hell and back, and all were eager to ease the journey for you and for others. They wish you the best of success in your own caregiving experiences, and they hope that by sharing some of what they wish they'd known, they will help make your cancer journey just a little easier. They were confident that you, too, will find your life enriched in unpredictable ways by your caregiving experience.

Finally, they all join me in hoping that we'll see a cancer-free world within our lifetimes.

# Acknowledgments

Even though an author's name is on the cover of a book, it takes many people to get a book into the reader's hands. The impetus to my writing **Things I Wish I'd Known** came from my maternal aunt, Marjorie Bram-MacPhillamy, who listened to my stories from Hope Lodge visits and said, "You must write a book." Now, more than five years later, I can show her the impact of her heartfelt appeal.

To fulfill my vision for this book, I needed access to a population of caregivers whose stories would represent a broad spectrum of geography, type of cancer, patient age, relationship of the caregiver to the patient, and duration of caregiving. This meant I needed to find and contact people I didn't yet know. Fortunately when both friends and strangers learned what I was doing, they quickly opened their memory banks, email directories, and phone books to speed me along.

Bryan Harter, LICSW, who manages the American Cancer Society's AstraZeneca Hope Lodge Center in Boston, confirmed that a book of this type was needed, posted invitations for guests to meet with me on a confidential basis to share their stories, and referred me to Bruce MacDonald, LICSW, an oncology social worker at Boston's world-renowned Dana-Farber Cancer Institute. Bruce offered his insights about the kinds of support caregivers need and generously wrote the preface to this book. I am deeply grateful to both of them.

Bryan also helped me connect with several other Hope Lodge managers who, in turn, posted the interview opportunity either in their lodges or in adjacent hospitals. These include Angela Putnam from the Hope Lodge Lois McClure-Bee Tabakin Building in Burlington, VT; Judy Mace of the Winn-Dixie Hope Lodge in Gainesville, Florida; Joleen Specht of the Marshfield Hope Lodge in Wisconsin; and Debra Aharonian of the Worcester Hope Lodge in Massachusetts. To all of them, my thanks.

Many of the friends I made during my years of volunteer leadership within ACS, both locally and nation-wide, also supported my networking to find interviewees. Among them, and they all deserve my heartfelt gratitude, were Steve Swanson, Cheryl McKenney, David Glidden, Kathleen Bond, Laura Hilderly, Janet Marcantonio, Bill Sherry, Carole Seigel, and Dr. Les Lockridge. Each of them either shared a personal caregiving story or referred others to me whose caregiving stories were compelling. Several of the Society's current or former staff members, including Marc Hymovitz and Kathy LeJeune, played similar roles. Finally, several local Relay For Life volunteers learned about my research and volunteered to be interviewed; those included Michele Genua, who proofread my first (very long!) draft. To these and other contributors whose names aren't explicitly cited here and whose insights weren't explicitly quoted in the book, I hope you know how grateful I will always be for your generous help.

Even clients and former professional colleagues chipped in. In particular, Paula Baker, now Chief Executive Officer for Freeman Health System in Joplin, Missouri, provided a caregiver referral; both she and her Board Executive Committee members offered invaluable moral support. Tom Casey, a former professional colleague, provided access to interviewees whose contributions were central to this book.

Every interviewee made a meaningful contribution, even if the interview wasn't quoted in the final manuscript. Some of the interviewees not only shared their stories, but also referred others to me whom they had met along the way. Those folks know who they are and how much I appreciate their ongoing support for this work. In particular, Rid Bullerjahn was not only an interviewee but gave generously of his time to "road test" the first edited draft and continued offering his marketing insights and networking on my behalf as the manuscript evolved. Mary Totten, a professional collaborator, offered both a compelling caregiver story and invaluable networking to help build the book's visibility and circulation.

Special thanks go to Dr. David Rosenthal, Dr. Andy Salner, Dr. Tracy Battaglia, and Don Gudaitis, each of whom read and offered either wise counsel or a testimonial on at least one version of the manuscript.

Finally, and certainly one of the most important people to thank, is my editor, Chris Angermann, President of Bardolf & Company, who brought his sharp mind and years of publishing experience to the task of pruning and focusing my work to help make it both interesting and user friendly. He convinced me that less is more.

As I've already said, no author produces a good book alone. Each of these individuals has left a meaningful fingerprint on this one and has earned my lasting appreciation.

For more information
or to contact the author,
go to

**www.thingsiwishidknown.com**

(Particularly useful may be
the Resources and Blog tabs.)

To contact the author, email

**thingsiwishidknown@gmail.com**